THE TRUTH ABOUT DIETARY SUPPLEMENTS

AN EVIDENCE-BASED GUIDE TO A SAFE MEDICINE CABINET

MAHTAB JAFARI

Author headshot by Navid Soheilian

Publishing services provided by 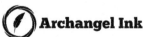 Archangel Ink

ISBN: 978-1-950043-33-0

To my husband, Rick, for being my rock.

To my mother, who inspired me to become a teacher and to have moral courage.

To my father, who instilled in me a sense of justice.

To our sons, Matin and Chris, who are my source of joy and pride.

And to my students, who remind me every day why I love teaching so much.

FOREWORD

A challenging question we healthcare providers get is: "Doctor, what nutritional supplement should I take?" We seldom have the answer, nor do we know how to find the best science. This book to our rescue!

In The Truth About Dietary Supplements, Dr. Jafari fills in the gaps in selecting smart supplements that health-conscious consumers are searching for. Thank you, Dr. Jafari! Not only does the author show us the science, but she also shows us her credentials. This book was literally written on the job. From a background of twenty-five years of teaching about dietary supplement and as a supplement researcher, her experience shines on every page. This riveting read, from the mind of a Doctor of Pharmacy, a Professor of Pharmaceutical Sciences, and a botanical scientist, takes readers on a journey through the wide world of supplement confusion and guides you on a path to make smart choices that are right for you. "Personalized Supplement Selection" is the current mantra of modern medicine.

Whenever I prescribe a dietary supplement for my patients or my family, I think show me the science, show me the safety, and show me the source. This book does all three.

As a show-me-the science reader and doctor I valued how each of her "Wow!" take-home points are supported by scientific references. And, for the reader who wishes a second helping of online scientific sources, these "Additional Resources "are highlighted at the end of each chapter.

For savvy readers who want to insert the right supplements into their daily diet, but just need a plan, this book is your plan. I highly recommend read it, do it, feel it and enjoy your path to vibrant health.

William Sears, MD; author, The Healthy Brain Book
San Clemente, California
June 2021

CONTENTS

PREFACE

First, I will say loud and clear, "I AM NOT AGAINST TAKING DIETARY SUPPLEMENTS." I used to take four supplements every day religiously. I began taking them because some deficiencies were detected in my blood and because of clear physiological signs. I was careful and responsible: I monitored their safety and made sure they did not interact with any other supplements or medications that I took. I also made sure that the supplements were of very high quality and were manufactured and sold by reputable companies who followed good manufacturing practices. Those supplements were part of optimizing my health. When I started writing this book, I was still taking these supplements, and I believed that this was necessary for me to remain healthy. But I have now stopped taking most of them. Why? At the end of this book I will tell you why, but for now I will keep you in suspense! A little bit of mystery is definitely a healthy thing for us all. ☺

Here is the most important idea in this book: *taking the right dietary supplements is good for us when we need them, but many people take supplements that they do not need and that are harming instead of helping them.* I wrote this book to share with you what I have learned about the dietary supplement industry over the past twenty-five years of teaching about it and researching pharmaceuticals and natural products in academia. My goal is to teach you how to choose and take the supplements that you truly need and avoid those that could cause you harm.

There is nothing that we want more than to take the best possible care of those around us, and during my career and training I have watched many, many people try to choose healthy lives for themselves and encourage those around them to do the same. When it comes to dietary supplements, most people are trying to do this all by themselves. They often have no guide, and usually they are unaware of the many risks and side effects of taking the wrong supplement. I wanted to provide a starting point, to give people a basic education—a roadmap—that will help them wisely navigate the many choices that confront them.

I grew up in a family who taught me at a very young age the value of education, service, and giving back to the community. My parents (and grandparents) raised me to be independent and outspoken, and to strive to live a purposeful life. I was born in Iran and lived there until I was about fifteen years old. As a young woman, I witnessed a revolution and the cruelties of war, and developed a strong sense of social justice and a passion for helping people in need. We immigrated twice: first to France, where I completed high school while learning French, and then to the U.S., where I had to learn English while attending college. I knew at a very young age what I wanted to do with my life. I loved science and teaching, and I was very interested in creating healthy communities. My grandmother had instilled a love of natural remedies in me. She taught me to eat fresh mint leaves to deal with an upset stomach and to take cinnamon during harsh winters to stay warm. She also believed that the remedy for headaches and impulsive eating was a handful of nuts. She always carried a bag of almonds and walnuts and would offer them to her family and friends—and even strangers—all day long. She used to say, "If you don't want to get sick, make sure to eat your nuts." She had her own garden where she grew fruits and vegetables, and she always kept a watchful eye on how the family was doing.

When I was sick as a child (in spite of eating all the nuts that my grandmother would force me to eat), my mother would take me to Dr. Maani. I still remember how painful my first strep throat infection was. I had a high fever and body aches and could not swallow anything, even my own saliva. Dr. Maani got a swab culture from my throat, checked it under his microscope, diagnosed me with a strep throat infection, and started me on antibiotics. He also recommended a warm saltwater gargle and a high dose of vitamin C. He would spend a lot of time explaining to me the importance of hand washing and building a strong immune system by eating fresh fruits and vegetables and sleeping at least eight hours every night. I loved to go back to Dr. Maani for follow-ups because the prize for getting better was always a lollipop made from fruit juice. In my neighborhood, Dr. Maani was considered a hero. Everyone respected and loved him. Many kids (including me) wanted to become Dr. Maani when we grew up. By now, you are probably thinking Dr. Maani was an amazing primary care physician, the neighborhood doctor who cared about his patients. Well, you are right in thinking that he was our neighborhood doctor, but he was not a physician. Dr. Maani was an amazing neighborhood pharmacist. He had a Pharm.D. (Doctor of Pharmacy) degree, a wealth of knowledge, an integrative approach to health, and a passion to help people. After completing my undergraduate studies (and learning English ☺), I went to the School of Pharmacy at the University of California in San Francisco (UCSF) to become a Dr. Maani. I graduated in 1994 and subsequently completed a clinical pharmacy residency program and joined the faculty at the UCSF School of Pharmacy.

I have been an educator, a scientist, and a healthcare provider for the past twenty-five years. Until 2005, the focus of my clinical and research activities was preventive medicine (how to prevent diseases from happening) and pharmacotherapy (choosing the right pharmaceuticals for the right disease). But in 2005, I shifted the focus of my research to slowing the aging process and improving healthspan. For the past fifteen years in my research laboratory at the University of California at Irvine, I have tested the impact of dietary supplements and botanical extracts on lifespan and healthspan, using various model systems such as cultured cells, fruit flies, and mice. The main goal of my research has been to delay aging and increase lifespan while improving healthspan. Throughout my career, my patients, friends, and family have asked me thousands of questions about dietary supplements. On a weekly basis I get questions via texts, emails, or phone calls from friends, family members, students, and the public about their dietary supplements. Some of these questions are presented in this book in the opening stories for each chapter. After years of answering these questions and, in some cases, preventing life-threatening disasters that were in danger of happening because of a dietary supplement, I decided to write this book.

I hope this book will educate my readers about the supplement industry, how to find out what supplements they need, how to make sure they are safe, and how to monitor them. I began to feel that writing this book was my duty and that educating the public about dietary supplements was a public health matter. Although over the years I have witnessed how dangerous and unsafe dietary supplements can be, I am not emotional when I talk about them. I present facts (and nothing but the facts). You should also know that I have no affiliation with any dietary supplement or pharmaceutical company. My research is not supported by any commercial entities, and although I am often invited to be a spokesperson for a nutritional or dietary supplement company, I never accept such invitations. I like my work and my research to be unbiased, and I take pride in having no conflict of interest.

Again, the purpose of this book is to educate the public about dietary supplements, but it is not meant to be an encyclopedia on supplements. Rather, it is intended as a very practical guidebook for how to navigate the world of dietary supplements and also to help you gain a framework for viewing your own health and nutritional choices. My goal is to teach you how to find the information you need and how to have a critical mind when it comes to your health.

This book is structured into seven chapters. Each chapter starts by telling a personal story, many of which spurred my research into dietary supplements, which is then followed by an investigation of the chapter's topic. Each chapter ends with two boxes: one that summarizes the major points of each chapter (Takeaways) and another that includes educational websites and further resources you may wish to explore (Additional Resources).

In chapter 1, "Dietary Supplements 101: A Few Basic Facts That We Should All Know," I talk about the industry in general: who are the makers and sellers of dietary supplements, what kind of economic trends we find (hint: this is an extremely lucrative and profitable industry!), and who is regulating the safety and quality of supplements (another hint: there is no pre-market or post-market testing of supplements!). The goal of this chapter is not to instill a fear of supplements in you, or to say that dietary supplements are unnecessary. Rather, the goal of this chapter and the entire book is *to help you to make informed decisions*.

In chapter 2, "Why Do We Need to Take Dietary Supplements?" I look at the reasons for taking supplements, and I also discuss the efficacy of traditional medical practices around the world, exploring how these can be very effective if practiced in the right context.

In chapter 3, "What's in That Pill? Is Your Dietary Supplement Safe?," I talk about the ingredients of dietary supplements and their safety. In this chapter, I argue that when it comes to dietary supplements, we need to be extra cautious, even more so than when we are taking pharmaceuticals, because the risks of dietary supplements are often hidden and unsuspected. That pill that we purchase without a prescription from a vitamin store or online may contain toxic ingredients, may be adulterated or spiked with prescription drugs, and may cause us serious harm.

In chapter 4, "The Science of Dietary Supplements," I talk about the challenges of interpreting the science or so-called science behind dietary supplements. In general, there is a large gap in the scientific literature when it comes to the use of dietary supplements; the flashy marketing claims of natural products often have no scientific backing.

In chapter 5, "The Power of Media to Brainwash the Public," I delve into the dangers caused by the media, magazines, social media platforms, and websites that claim to be teaching us about what is "healthy." I also talk about the marketing practices used by supplement companies and the psychology of celebrity influencers, which have a shockingly large impact on health and nutrition trends.

In chapter 6, "The Truth about Pet Supplements," I talk about the ever-expanding market for pet supplements and the lack of scientific evidence on the safety and efficacy of these products to actually improve pet well-being.

In chapter 7, "Learning How to Take the Dietary Supplements You Need," I give you the questions you need to ask yourself and your healthcare providers to get you the right answers about your body's needs and how to choose the right dietary supplements. I also explain how to find a trustworthy dietary supplement manufacturer and how to monitor for the safety of the supplements you take.

And finally, in the Appendix, "Dietary Supplements and COVID-19," I talk about the scientific evidence on dietary supplements to combat COVID-19.

I hope that after reading this book you will be a more informed, savvy consumer, able to be discerning about dietary supplements and to see through clever marketing and dangerous health trends that might steal both your money and your health. I also hope that you will share the knowledge that you have learned with your family and friends.

To your health!

Mahtab Jafari

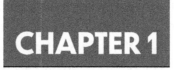

CHAPTER 1

DIETARY SUPPLEMENTS 101:
A FEW BASIC FACTS THAT WE SHOULD ALL KNOW

STORY

My cousin began taking dietary supplements when she turned forty, and she quickly became an enthusiastic connoisseur. She had all kinds of products to recommend for her friends and family and declared that she felt better than ever since beginning her new dietary-supplements-enriched life. I became curious, and one day I asked her to show me all the supplements that she was taking. She pulled open a drawer that was packed full of about twenty bottles of various sizes and colors. Even though I knew she was "into" supplements, I was still a little taken aback at the sheer number of them.

I looked at the labels and recognized most of what she was taking as quite common, but there were a few esoteric items as well. When I asked how she had found these more exotic supplements, she explained that she had discovered them based on her own research. Later, I would learn that most of her "research" was a mix of popular magazine articles, TV advertisements, and the advice of a salesperson in her local health food store. She had never taken a blood test to determine if her body was actually deficient in any of the vitamins or minerals that she was faithfully swallowing every day. She had never consulted a scientific journal article to see if the dosages of the herbs she was taking were excessive and potentially harmful if mixed with other supplements and medications.

A little probing revealed that my cousin was spending nearly $700 a month, or $8,400 per year, on this cocktail of dietary supplements! Even though the cost was so significant, it was increasingly clear to me as we spoke that she did not know what effect these supplements were having on her. Maybe the supplements were helping her, but it was hard to tell: she is a healthy and happy woman who neither smokes nor drinks, exercises regularly, and eats a balanced diet—all lifestyle practices that are proven to offer the best health benefits. However, if you asked her, that drawer full of supplements was the secret behind her health.

What is the truth of the matter? Were these supplements a worthwhile investment in her future health, as she believed? Or was she paying thousands of dollars to feel as if she were taking good care of herself, but not actually receiving any true benefits? Though my cousin's case may be extreme, she is part of a growing trend: Americans are spending more money on dietary supplements than ever before in the belief that it will make them healthier and happier. Is their money well spent?

How can health-conscious consumers find out what (if any) supplements they need to improve their health? And how can they test the quality, safety, and efficacy of the dietary supplements that they consider taking? The goal of this book is to answer these questions and equip you with an understanding of what supplements are and how they work, the ins and outs of government regulation of the supplement industry, and the specific questions and tests that can help you to get your body everything it needs and nothing that it does not.

DIETARY SUPPLEMENTS

First things first: what exactly is a dietary supplement?

The idea is a very simple one: dietary supplements are meant to supplement our diets! If certain foods are scarce, or a person has difficulty absorbing a particular nutrient, supplements can be taken to remediate that deficiency.

The supplements available today can be grouped into different families, according to the kind of nutrient they are providing. Throughout this book, when I refer to a dietary supplement, I am talking about one of the following:

- **Vitamins.** These are essential nutrients that the body cannot make itself but which it needs in order to grow. There are thirteen vitamins: A, C, D, E, K, and a group of eight B vitamins (thiamin, riboflavin, niacin, pantothenic acid, biotin, B6, B12, and folate). Of these, only vitamins D and K can be made by our bodies under the right circumstances; the rest we must gain from our diet and are often sold in the form of supplements. (See the Additional Resources box at the end of this chapter for more information on each vitamin's function and what foods contain them.)

- **Minerals.** Our bodies also require certain minerals, such as calcium or sodium, which must be obtained through the foods we eat. Unlike vitamins, though, minerals are inorganic. They are not produced by the plants themselves, but instead are absorbed into plants from the soil.

- **Herbs and Botanicals.** This category is extremely wide, including any plant-based supplement that might offer some particular health benefit. These herbal remedies were the earliest form of medicine. Willow bark is a perfect example. For over a thousand years, it was used as a pain reliever in many cultures. Eventually, the active molecule in willow bark was isolated and reproduced synthetically and sold as you and I know it today: aspirin.

- **Proteins.** This grouping can be produced by either animals or plants. It was at first marketed to the elite fitness industry and taken by body builders and extreme athletes. Protein supplements focus on increasing the amount of essential amino acids (the building blocks of proteins) and proteins in a person's diet. These performance-enhancing supplements have become widely popular, even though the average American's diet already provides adequate amounts of protein.

- **Probiotics and Enzymes.** Probiotics—live microorganisms that are often found in fermented foods such as yogurt—aid in digestion, and enzymes are organic substances that catalyze chemical reactions. Our digestive system breaks down carbohydrates, fats, and proteins with the help of systemic and digestive enzymes as well as live bacteria and yeasts. We need the right amounts of these enzymes and good bacteria in our bodies in order to easily process and absorb necessary nutrients.

These different families of dietary supplements are packaged and sold to us in many forms and combinations: as pills, powders, gels, energy bars, and teas. Some are also offered as shots, such as vitamin B12. Generally, these products are marketed as something like a cross between a "superfood" and "nature's medicine." They claim to be able to help the body do all kinds of things: protect against memory loss, bolster the immune system, increase bone density, calm anxiety, enhance sexual performance, and, of course, help us lose weight. For every problem (or potential problem), health stores have aisles full of supplements that promise to save the day.

DIETARY SUPPLEMENTS ARE BIG BUSINESS

Over the past ten years, people have been steadily spending more and more money on supplements. In 2017, $40 billion dollars were made from the sales of these supplements in the United States. The industry's growth rate has been phenomenal: In 1994, there were 4,000 dietary supplement products on the American market. In 2017, there were over 80,000 (Pew, 2017). This is a 2000% increase (yes, two thousand percent) in thirty-three years!

The majority of Americans report taking some form of dietary supplements daily. Most take multivitamins, which have long been the staple of the industry, but enormous growth has appeared in the sale of supplements that claim to boost energy and act as performance enhancers for athletes (often labeled as "sports nutrition") and also those marketed as weight-loss aids (Zion, 2017). In 2016, the National Center for Health Statistics of the Centers for Disease Control and Prevention completed one of the largest surveys of American spending on health to date. They reported that the public spent $30 billion dollars on complementary health approaches and that nearly 60 million Americans spent money out of pocket to either visit a complementary health practitioner or purchase supplements made from natural products (National Institutes of Health [NIH], 2016). *Consumer Research Surveys* estimates that these numbers are likely to increase as health-conscious Americans who are already taking multivitamins now also report that they are regularly taking additional supplements. In addition, the survey found that young Americans who regularly purchased supplements reported that they expect to begin taking more over the next ten years (Council for Responsible Nutrition, 2015).

This is all very good news for companies that produce and sell dietary supplements. The trends in sales are inspiring tiny startup manufacturers to open up for business and tempting colossal established companies to dip their toes in the water as well. The profit margins on supplement products can be wildly high. Because something like calcium is cheap and plentiful and takes very little investment to purify and prepare for consumption, the cost of the product to the producer for each bottle is about five cents, while the consumer's cost may be $9.99, more than a 1000% markup (GNC, 2019).

Investors smell a profit and are following their noses: In 2017, Amazon.com introduced its own line of vitamins. In 2018, another giant, Nestlé, long a superstar in the American candy and food market, sold off part of its candy holdings and is reportedly looking to reinvest by buying up supplement manufacturers (Dewey, 2018). A bit further afield, Clorox, known for its household cleaning supplies, broke into the industry by offering to buy the supplement manufacturer Nutranext for $700 million dollars in 2018 (Lombardo, 2018).

Globally, it is estimated that the supplement industry is worth an astonishing $132 billion dollars (Zion, 2017). It is estimated that this number will more than double in five years. The top supplement firms are based in the United States, but their reach is becoming global. Herbalife, a major American supplement manufacturer, has recently dedicated $90 million to expanding their presence in China, where they are working to capture the attention of middle-class consumers (Y. Wu, 2018). In 2018, GNC had 40% of its shares sold to a Chinese pharmaceutical company, which obtained exclusive rights to distribute GNC products on the Chinese market (K. Wu, 2018). All of this stock shuffling and these giant mergers are going to continue. Major companies are positioning themselves for the windfall that they know is coming as worldwide demand for supplements increases. Yet despite the dietary supplement industry's continued growth, it is not required to follow the same regulatory standards that the pharmaceuticals industry does.

DIETARY SUPPLEMENTS ARE NOT REGULATED LIKE PHARMACEUTICALS

But what does this astronomical growth in the supplement industry mean for the health of the people who are buying their products? Does an increase in the production and consumption of dietary supplements mean that we are all becoming healthier and healthier? Who is monitoring supplement manufacturing? Who is checking for the safety and efficacy of supplements before they hit the market?

The short answer is: nobody! Although there are many different kinds of supplements, from prenatal vitamins to protein bars to sexual enhancement teas, what they all have in common is their legal classification as dietary supplements, which gives them a free pass on pre-market testing. They are not sold or regulated in the same manner as pharmaceuticals, which are subject to years of scientific testing, clinical trials, and manufacturing quality assurance before they are eligible to be approved by the Food and Drug Administration (FDA) and made available to the public. Even with these rigorous requirements, many pharmaceuticals have been removed from the market due to adverse effects that were not observed during testing (or, more nefariously, not reported). However, any product that is sold as a dietary supplement can jump right onto health food or grocery store shelves without undergoing any testing and without meeting any burden of proof for its claims to the FDA (Scott, 2015).

For comparison's sake, let's see what it takes for a new pharmaceutical to make it onto the market.

While many pharmaceutical companies spend much of their time selling slight variations of already-approved drugs, the process of testing and gaining approval for a new medication is uncertain, time-intensive, and very expensive, as we will see below. This leads to what we call a "high barrier to entry": because of the great cost involved, generally only pharmaceutical giants can manufacture and sell new drugs. How high is this barrier? Out of five thousand candidate drugs, on average only *one* will eventually be given FDA approval and subsequently be sold to the public (Angell, 2005).

The initial stage of pharmaceutical development is called "discovery." Drugs are developed in response to a specific disease or condition. By carefully studying a disease, researchers hope to identify what chain of events at the molecular level is harming the body. If they can isolate and understand that chain, they can look for ways to break it or reverse its effects. This discovery phase often takes place in federally funded or private academic institutions, or within a handful of smaller startup pharmaceutical and biotechnology companies. It is usually the composite work of many scientists, and it can take years, even decades, for this research to lead to a possible drug candidate or cure.

Once a potential cure is in sight, the role of pharmaceutical companies usually grows. Academic institutions and independent researchers are not equipped to perform large clinical trials or to manufacture and sell drugs, and do not have the funding to support the developmental stages of preparing a new drug. Only well-established private companies can manufacture, run clinical trials for, market, and distribute drugs.

In 1962, the FDA raised the threshold for the requirements to put a drug on the market. New pharmaceuticals had to be proven to be not only safe but also effective. This led to two stages of testing required of all new drugs: pre-clinical trials and clinical trials. In the pre-clinical investigation stage, all the potential drug candidates that match the criteria for combatting the condition are sorted through and tested in animal models to identify those that will be the safest and most efficacious. Thousands of drug candidates fail to pass this part of the investigation phase.

A very few candidate drugs will survive to the next round of development: clinical testing on human subjects. This is expensive and, obviously, a very high-risk undertaking. Indeed, a major task of pharmaceutical companies is recruiting human subjects for these clinical trials. Finally, the FDA reviews these trials and determines whether the drug meets the threshold for safety and efficacy and merits their approval for public consumption.

How long does all this take? The pre-clinical trials, clinical trials, and FDA review process for a new drug requires on average six to ten years to complete, and the cost of development is anywhere from $100 million to $800 million (Angell, 2005). Yet, despite this expensive and arduous process to protect public health, adverse effects that were not observed (or not fully disclosed) during the investigational and clinical testing still do occur after pharmaceuticals are put on the market. This is partially due to the fact that people with medical conditions that were excluded from the clinical trial are able to take the drug once it is approved. The bottom line is that the system is far from perfect, but it has delivered a relatively strong form of safety and quality control for pharmaceuticals.

In sum, because of the length and expense of this regulatory process, and the lingering possibility of failure, the mass manufacture and sale of pharmaceuticals is usually controlled by those senior companies that already have the millions necessary to fund the clinical trials that are required to gain FDA approval.

How does the story of pharmaceuticals relate to dietary supplements? Because supplements are treated as a wholly different category under federal law, *there is no similar regulatory process for them.*

This became especially important after 1994, when the FDA widened the definition of dietary supplements to be more inclusive. Instead of referring mostly to straightforward vitamin and mineral supplements, now the government considered all products that contained "a vitamin, a mineral, an herb or other botanical, an amino acid, [or] a dietary substance" and were intended to "supplement the diet" to be dietary supplements (FDA, 2016). The floodgates were opened: Hundreds of products that would have been classified as drugs could now be sold as dietary supplements. FDA regulations only mandate correct labeling, requiring that the "identity, purity, strength, and composition of dietary supplement products are accurate," the same standards expected of food (Pew, 2017).

The effect of the legislation was immediate. To offer one example, between 1990 and 1997, herbal supplement use increased by 380% in the United States (Eisenberg et al., 1998), in great part because so many manufacturers were putting new products on the market under the revised guidelines. Because of the very low level of federal oversight, it is relatively cheap for anyone to develop and sell new products. This "low barrier to entry" means that many small companies of very different quality and experience are selling supplements (which are also of varied quality!) (Sax, 2015). What has developed is an industry that is both immensely profitable and highly unaccountable, a "Wild West" for the health sector.

In 2015, the FDA performed random complete quality control inspections on only 500 of the nearly 13,000 registered manufacturers of supplements in the U.S. They found violations of good manufacturing practices in more than half of the 500 that were spot-checked. Violations included producers' failure to accurately label their products, contamination issues, and inadequate quality control and measurement of ingredients (Pew, 2017). The cold hard fact is that the vast majority of U.S. supplement manufacturers and the large number of foreign companies who sell on U.S. markets are subject to no outside review of their products before they are available to consumers, and only a small percentage of companies are being checked for basic quality control each year.

So what would it take for the government to force a dietary supplement off of the market? How does the system identify dangerous or faulty supplements? We know that the FDA does not require that supplements be tested before being sold, so the obvious and unfortunate answer is that *the testing happens on the consumers,* and it is the consumers who have the responsibility of identifying dangerous and faulty supplements.

The FDA will step in to recall a product only *after* it has caused serious damage to the public. This is not because the FDA is negligent, but merely a reflection of the fact that the FDA is understaffed and underfunded. The companies that make the products are supposed to report to the FDA when consumers report serious adverse effects to them. This places most of the responsibility for policing a product in the hands of the very people who are making money from selling that product—an accountability nightmare.

An acute example of this problem occurred in 2013, when a weight-loss aid called OxyElitePro, produced by USP Labs and sold through GNC, was found to be the cause of hepatitis in twenty-nine people, leading to severe liver damage. The FDA found the link by connecting the dots of multiple adverse event reports and subsequently forced GNC to pull the product from the market—but only after it caused one death and multiple users needed liver transplants (FDA Criminal Investigations, 2016).

The existing legislation on dietary supplements creates a system in which the government must put out one blazing fire after the next. Steven Tave, the director of the FDA's Office of Dietary Supplements Program, faces a gigantic and frustrating task, working with a staff of only twenty-six people and a budget of $5 million. In his mind, when Congress passed the Dietary Supplement Health Education Act in 1994, the bill still made sense. In 1994, there were about 4,000 dietary supplements on the market, manufactured by about 600 companies for a total revenue of about $4 billion. In 2017, about 80,000 dietary supplements were produced by 6,000 companies. "The products we see today have gone way beyond that sort of core group that they were in 1994," said Tave. "Now they're promoted for all sorts of things—some are long term, some are short term, some are chemicals no one's ever seen before. It's a much different universe than it was at the time" (Brodwin, 2017).

The FDA's Office of Dietary Supplements Program does not have sufficient resources to monitor the safety of dietary supplements. In most cases, this office learns about the harmful effects of a supplement only after it has harmed people. In a presentation at the American Herbal Products Association's 7th Annual Botanical Congress, Tave highlighted recent collaborations between the FDA and the responsible supplement industry. His presentation talked about the top three Office of Dietary Supplements Program priorities: safety, product integrity, and informed decision-making. It is reassuring to know that responsible manufacturers of dietary supplements are looking for ways to not only comply with the law's requirements but also to set higher standards for the entire industry.

I could not agree more with Steven Tave. I have worked closely with FDA officials and investigators on developing educational programs for my students and initiatives to ensure public safety. Two of these programs earned us awards because the projects my students developed were selected to be implemented nationwide. I have also attended public presentations by FDA investigators on their work in issuing injunction and seizure letters to insufficiently responsible dietary supplement firms. I have seen firsthand how understaffed the FDA is and how hard FDA investigators try to ensure public safety with only limited resources. My hope is that more dietary supplement companies will join the "responsible supplement industry" and that the FDA will be allocated more resources to ensure the safety of the consumers who take dietary supplements.

Although many organizations who lobby for dietary supplements claim that FDA regulates the supplements, below is what is listed on the FDA website (FDA, 2019). The first sentence—"FDA regulates both finished dietary supplements products and dietary ingredients"— has been used out of context by a number of supporters of the dietary supplements industry without including the entire statement. I have underlined and bolded the sentences that emphasize the fact that FDA does not evaluate and regulate the safety and efficacy of the dietary supplements the way it does for pharmaceuticals prior to entering the market:

FDA regulates both finished dietary supplement products and dietary ingredients. ***FDA regulates dietary supplements under a different set of regulations than those covering "conventional" foods and drug products****. Under the Dietary Supplement Health and Education Act of 1994 (DSHEA):*

- *Manufacturers and distributors of dietary supplements and dietary ingredients are prohibited from marketing products that are adulterated or misbranded.* ***That means that these firms are responsible for evaluating the safety and labeling of their products before marketing to ensure that they meet all the requirements of DSHEA and FDA regulations****.*

- *FDA is responsible for taking action against any adulterated or misbranded dietary supplement product* ***after it reaches the market****.*

In summary, according to the FDA, "The U.S. Food and Drug Administration (FDA) does not have the authority to review dietary supplement products for safety and effectiveness before they are marketed" (FDA, 2017).

MISSING NUMBERS: RESEARCH EXPENDITURES ON DIETARY SUPPLEMENTS

As we saw in the beginning of this chapter, there are ample data to prove how profitable the dietary supplement industry is becoming. More elusive, however, are the numbers that tell us the amount that these companies spend on researching the safety and efficacy of the products that they are selling all over the world. Most supplement companies are anxious to keep their spending habits on research a secret, and the law allows them to—a privilege not enjoyed by pharmaceutical companies, which are obligated by federal law to disclose at least some of their numbers to the public.

For a variety of reasons that we will explore, research is a low priority for most supplement producers: the lion's share of their budgets goes to brand formation and marketing. Marketing is of critical importance for supplements sales because most people purchase a particular product based on word of mouth. Prescription drugs come to us through the order of a physician, but supplements are usually chosen without any input from a healthcare provider, with some exceptions. Customers choose products based on their own intuition about what they think they need and what they believe a certain supplement will do for them. Informal marketing tactics, such as blogs, celebrity endorsements, and health information websites that tout a product's wonderful (if unproven) benefits, are essential for the kind of grassroots discovery process that leads people to supplements. Appealing labeling and branding is critical for sales because first impressions are vital (no plain orange bottles with tiny font on them here!). In short, while dietary supplement products are multiplying rapidly along with the formation of giant marketing engines to promote them, the research on their safety and efficacy lags further and further behind. Although there are more and more bottles to choose from, in many cases, very few studies are being undertaken to prove the value and safety of what is in them.

To put this in perspective, consider the case of "Big Pharma." The pharmaceutical industry is often lambasted for its own massive expenditures on marketing, and rightly so. Critics claim that pharmaceutical companies spend nearly as much on marketing their products to the public as they do on research (Angell, 2005). Big Pharma has a lot of weight to throw around, but a close look reveals that the dietary supplement industry is even more shocking in its lopsided spending patterns. While pharmaceutical industry sales ($450 billion in 2017) dwarf that of the supplement sector ($40 million), dietary supplement companies spend *far more* on marketing than on research (if they commit to *any* research at all). As we will see, this is because of the very different legal restraints that guide the two industries.

So how much do we know about the safety and usefulness of the dietary supplements that we buy? Who is researching the actual effects of these products on our health?

Independent research on the efficacy of dietary supplements is growing, but very slowly in comparison with the market. The U.S. FDA added dietary supplements to its research agenda for the first time in 1994, but less than 10% of the nutrition-related projects undertaken since then had to do with supplement use (Kuchler & Toole, 2015). This research is often publicly funded and performed in academic institutions. The most important potential sponsor of this research is the National Institutes of Health (NIH), which is funded by the U.S. government and is the world's largest coordinator of biomedical and health research (investing almost $40 billion annually in research).

It is only relatively recently, however, that the NIH has started systematically researching dietary supplements. In 1995, the Office of Dietary Supplements (ODS) was created within the NIH. This small branch of the NIH is tasked with coordinating projects related to the safety and efficacy of dietary supplements. In 2011, the NIH invested $249 million dollars in supplement research—just 0.8% of the total NIH budget. In that same year, ODS committed $10.2 million dollars to research (NIH, 2017). This is much better than thirty years ago, when there was no designated office for investigating supplements and no systematic approach to researching dietary supplements as a distinct category. But this research budget is still small potatoes in the world of medical research.

A tremendous variety of substances are labeled as dietary supplements, and a myriad of different health claims are attached to them. With such a limited budget, only a handful of substances and their properties can be rigorously tested. In 2012, the dietary supplement projects funded by NIH were clustered into several dominant categories: studies related to cancer (61%), cardiovascular disease (47%), and women's reproductive health (38%). As far as which ingredients were most studied, botanicals (22%), vitamins (20%), and lipids (14%) were the top three categories (Garcia-Cazarin et al., 2014). This is encouraging progress, but there is a pressing need for greater funding and expanded research agendas. The ODS itself warns consumers about this dearth of research: "Although vitamin and mineral supplements have been available for decades, their health effects have been the subject of detailed scientific research only within the last 15–20 years" (NIH, 2019).

It is unlikely that federally funded research alone can ever close this gap. The companies profiting from supplement sales must use their resources to invest in studies that will protect their customers. Fortunately, many dietary supplement companies have a conscience and are dedicated to supporting the health of those who put faith in their products. These companies gain certification from independent review agencies such as U.S. Pharmacopeia, and they commit to good manufacturing practices and sound research and development goals.

Over time, the research of such companies will add to our knowledge of how to use supplements wisely and safely.

But, of course, many dietary supplement producers will not voluntarily undertake this research. A rapidly growing industry that promises high profit margins is a tempting proposition. The market encourages companies to meet consumer demand by selling more supplement products that claim to help us, but there is little incentive for those companies to substantiate their claims by investing in careful research and clinical trials. The FDA does not require companies to prove that dietary supplement products are effective before they put them on the market, in stark contrast with the pre-market testing of pharmaceuticals. This is the fundamental problem for you and me as consumers: How do we know if what is being sold to us as a health aid is truly good for our health?

CONCLUSION

Ironically, the average American probably has a lot more confidence in products labeled as dietary supplements than does the director of the FDA's ODS. In a survey of American adults, "about 50% reported that dietary supplements that aid weight loss must be approved by a government agency for safety and efficacy before they can be sold to consumers." In a smaller sample of 185 undergraduate students, "about 75% erroneously believed that the FDA was responsible for ensuring the safety of supplements before they could be sold and nearly 50% believed the content of dietary supplements is analyzed by the FDA" (Dodge, 2016).

The marketing messages of supplement manufacturers have successfully created a strong positive bias in favor of supplements: people associate supplements with health. Supplements are able to get a free ride off the credibility of pharmaceuticals, with many people assuming that supplements meet that high level of product control and testing that prescription drugs must reach.

And so, people continue to walk down the long aisles of dietary supplements found in nearly every grocery store and confidently buy the products, assuming that the health benefits reported on their labels are all accurate. Only in the smallest of print, so tiny that we need a magnifying glass to read it, do we find the one thing that we absolutely know to be true about supplements: "These statements have not been evaluated by the Food and Drug Administration."

TAKEAWAYS

- Vitamins, minerals, herbs and botanicals, proteins, probiotics, and enzymes are all considered to be dietary supplements, and are sold in many different forms.

- Vitamins are essential nutrients that our bodies require but cannot produce themselves. Some minerals are also essential. These must be obtained through our diet.

- The sale and consumption of dietary supplements is on the rise: There are over 80,000 dietary supplements on the American market today, and $40 billion dollars were made on supplement sales in the U.S. in 2017.

- The global dietary supplement industry is worth $132 billion dollars and by 2022 is projected to reach $232 billion dollars.

- Despite this growth, there is a stunning deficit in the research behind these products and in their safety and efficacy.

- The FDA does not require that dietary supplements meet any pre-market testing to prove that they are effective and safe, as it does with pharmaceuticals. Instead, the FDA will only investigate a dietary supplement once consumers have reported enough adverse events to its office.

ADDITIONAL RESOURCES

- A basic overview of vitamins and minerals and good food sources for each:

  Harvard Health Publishing: Listing of Vitamins.

  https://www.health.harvard.edu/staying-healthy/listing_of_vitamins

- Consumer surveys on supplement use in the United States:

  Council for Responsible Nutrition and Pew Charitable Trusts.

  https://www.crnusa.org/

- Information on the regulation of supplements: Office of Dietary Supplements Program.

  https://www.fda.gov/food/dietarysupplements/

- Information on dietary supplement recalls: Food and Drug Administration Recalls.

  https://www.fda.gov/food/recallsoutbreaksemergencies/recalls/

- Information on NIH-funded studies on dietary supplements: Computer Access to Research on Dietary Supplements (CARDS) Database.

  https://ods.od.nih.gov/Research/CARDS_Database.aspx

REFERENCES

Angell, M. (2005). *The truth about drug companies: How they deceive us and what to do about it.* Random House.

Brodwin, E. (2017). *A batch of contaminated supplements has been recalled— Here's how the products get into stores.* Business Insider Nordic. http:// nordic.businessinsider.com/dangerous-supplements-vitamins-in -stores-2017-8/

Council for Responsible Nutrition. (2015). *The dietary supplement consumer.* http://www.crnusa.org/CRN-consumersurvey-archives/2015/

Dewey, C. (2018, January 17). Why Nestle sold its U.S. candy business— And bought a vitamin company. *The Washington Post.* https://www .washingtonpost.com/news/wonk/wp/2018/01/17/why-nestle-sold -its-u-s-candy-business-and-bought-a-vitamin-company

Dodge, T. (2016). Consumers' perceptions of the dietary supplement health and education act: Implications and recommendations. *Drug Testing and Analysis 8*(3–4), 407–9.

Eisenberg, D.M., Davis, R.B., Ettner, S.L., et al. (1998). Trends in alternative medicine use in the United States, 1990–1997: Results of a follow-up national survey. *JAMA, 280*(18),1569–1575. doi:10.1001 /jama.280.18.1569

Food and Drug Administration. (2016, August). *Dietary supplements: New dietary ingredients notifications and related issues: Guidance for industry.* https://www.fda.gov/media/99538/download

Food and Drug Administration. (2017, November). *What you need to know about dietary supplements.* https://www.fda.gov/food/buy-store-serve -safe-food/what-you-need-know-about-dietary-supplements

Food and Drug Administration (2019, August). *Dietary supplements.* https://www.fda.gov/food/dietary-supplements

Food and Drug Administration Criminal Investigations. (2016, December). *GNC enters into agreement with Department of Justice to improve its practices and keep potentially illegal dietary supplements out of the marketplace.* Department of Health and

Human Services, Food and Drug Administration. https://
www.fda.gov/iceci/criminalinvestigations/ucm533077.htm

Garcia-Cazarin, M.L., Wambogo, E.A., Regan, K.S. & Davis, C.D.
(2014). Dietary supplement research portfolio at the NIH, 2009-
2011. *The Journal of Nutrition, 144*(4), 414–8. https://www.ncbi.nlm
.nih.gov/pmc/articles/PMC3952619/

General Nutrition Centers. (2019, September 15). Product Page, GNC
Calcium Plus 1000. https://www.gnc.com/calcium/066222.html

Kuchler, F. & Toole, A.A. (2015, June 1). *Federal support for nutrition research
trends upward as USDA share declines*. Department of Health and
Human Services, Food and Drug Administration. https://www.ers
.usda.gov/amber-waves/2015/june/federal-support-for-nutrition
-research-trends-upward-as-usda-share-declines

Lombardo, C. (2018, March 12). Clorox to buy dietary-supplement
maker Nutranext for $700 million. *The Wall Street Journal*. https://
www.wsj.com/articles/clorox-to-buy-dietary-supplement-maker
-nutranext-for-700-million-1520862995

National Institutes of Health. (2016). *Americans spend $30 billion a year out of
pocket on complementary health approaches*. U.S. Department of Health and
Human Services, National Institutes of Health. https://nccih.nih.gov
/research/results/spotlight/americans-spend-billions

———.(2017). *NIH Office of Dietary Supplements: Strategic plan 2017–2021*.
U.S. Department of Health and Human Services, National
Institutes of Health. https://ods.od.nih.gov/pubs/strategicplan
/ODSStrategicPlan2017-2021.pdf

———. (2019). *Estimates of funding for various research, condition, and disease
categories (RCDC)*. U.S. Department of Health and Human Services,
National Institutes of Health. https://report.nih.gov/categorical
_spending.aspx

Pew Charitable Trusts. (2017, October 24). *Dietary supplements: What are
they and how are they regulated?* http://www.pewtrusts.org/en/research
-and-analysis/fact-sheets/2017/10/dietary-supplements-what-are
-they-and-how-are-they-regulated

Sax, J.K. (2015). Dietary supplements are not all safe and not all food: How the low cost of dietary supplements preys on the consumer. *American Journal of Law & Medicine, 41*(2–3). 374–394. doi:10.1177/0098858815591523

Scott, C. (2015, March 26). *Americans are wasting billions of dollars every year on health supplements that don't even work.* Business Insider. http://www.businessinsider.com/money-wasted-on-health-supplements-2015-3.

Wu, K. (2018, February 13). *China's Harbin Pharma to buy stake in U.S. health retailer GNC.* Reuters. https://www.reuters.com/article/us-gnc-harbin-pharma-investment/chinas-harbin-pharma-to-buy-stake-in-u-s-health-retailer-gnc-idUSKCN1FY0DL

Wu, Y. (2018, February 13). *Herbalife launches $90m fund to accelerate China growth.* China Money Network. https://www.chinamoneynetwork.com/2018/02/13/herbalife-launches-90m-china-growth-impact-investment-fund

Zion Market Research. (2017, January 4). *Global dietary supplements market is expected to reach around USD 220.3 billion in 2022.* Zion Market Research. https://www.zionmarketresearch.com/news/dietary-supplements-market

CHAPTER 2

WHY DO WE NEED TO TAKE DIETARY SUPPLEMENTS?

STORY

In 2014, within a four-month period, I had two knee injuries from skiing. On both knees I developed bone bruises, and on the left one I also developed a Baker's cyst. The traumas that caused these injuries were not dramatic; I certainly did not walk away with any exciting stories to impress my friends with. The first was simply due to over-extending my leg while going down the slope and hitting a rope. Yet, mundane as they were, each injury took almost six months to heal.

That summer, I went to see a new physician, an MD who also practiced integrative medicine. She ordered a blood test to evaluate my nutritional status. At first, I put the test off. I knew that I ate a pretty healthy diet, and I was not sure it was really necessary or pertinent to my knee injuries. The test was not cheap, and it was not covered by my health insurance, either—another reason to drag my feet. But I eventually did the blood test, and that was one of the best decisions I have ever made.

Among other things, I discovered that I had very low levels of vitamin D, low enough to put me in the "very" deficient category. I was surprised because I spend a lot of time in the outdoors. This deficiency explained the weakness that perhaps made me more vulnerable to my knee injuries and also why it took so long for them to heal. When we become adults, our bones are no longer growing, but new bone tissue is constantly replacing the old. Severe vitamin D deficiency can interfere with the formation of new bone tissue and delay it. Although current published studies provide no conclusive recommendations on the benefits of vitamin D for bone healing, in response to my low vitamin D levels, I immediately started taking vitamin D supplements.

The test also showed that I was low in coenzyme Q10, magnesium, and eicosapentaenoic acid (EPA), which is a long-chain omega-3 fatty acid that is harder for the body to produce as it ages. I started taking CoQ10, EPA, and magnesium dietary supplements every day. All of these nutrients play an important role in maintaining the body's homeostasis. If I had continued to be deficient in these substances, over time I would have left my body more susceptible to injury and illness. I eventually modified my diet so that it was rich in seafood and green leafy vegetables and stopped taking some of the above dietary supplements. Three months after being on this new diet and off supplements, I had another blood test, and my levels for vitamin D, CoQ10, and EPA were normal.

DIETARY SUPPLEMENTS CAN BE GOOD FOR US

The first chapter of this book waved a giant red flag, warning potential consumers that the dietary supplement industry has grown exponentially, producing more and more health products whose claims are often based on inadequate research, and whose quality is subject to hardly any regulation. This should make us very cautious, but it should not overshadow an age-old truth: **In the right dose and under the right circumstances, high-quality dietary supplements can truly be good for us.**

Science and experience tell the same story: Our bodies need the right nutritional balance in order to be well. Though we should receive this balance primarily through our diets, in some cases, such as my own, it is helpful and even essential to get these nutrients from dietary supplements as well.

In chapter 7, I will discuss how to detect particular deficiencies you might have and how to verify that the supplements you buy are trustworthy products. In this chapter, however, we will consider more broadly some key questions about our nutritional needs and the usefulness of supplements in different cases:

- What role have supplements played in overcoming malnutrition?
- Should we be concerned that food might be less nutritious today than it used to be, as some claim?
- How do our nutritional needs change as we age?

Once we have considered all these questions, we will also look at the ways in which traditional and complementary medicine have been used to support overall health and treat specific ailments for centuries.

HISTORICAL PERSPECTIVE: DISCOVERY, INVENTION, AND THE ROLES OF DIETARY SUPPLEMENTS IN COMBATTING MALNUTRITION

For much of human history, most people were deficient in particular vitamins or minerals. The exact deficiencies varied according to time and place, but malnutrition's effects were often devastating and drastically shortened lives. Dietary supplements were originally developed to combat this pervasive problem.

It was in the early twentieth century that scientists and physicians began trying to isolate the compounds within food, using the term "vitamin" to describe those *vital*, literally "life-giving," substances that they found. Prior to 1900, germ theory was the most common explanation for every health problem. Disease, not deficiency, was perceived to be the culprit behind most human physical woes. Linking certain conditions to a lack of a particular vitamin rather than an infection was a bold proposition. To prove that this was so, scientists needed to identify the chemical structure of vitamins to demonstrate their necessity to human health. The existence of vitamins was an astonishing discovery: the building blocks of food and the secrets of nutrition could be seen for the first time (Semba, 2012).

In the 1930s, the first experiments were undertaken to put a vitamin in pill form. Hungarian researcher Albert Szent-Györgyi successfully isolated and identified ascorbic acid, which was the necessary nutrient to prevent scurvy, the mysterious affliction affecting so many sailors deprived for months at a time of fresh fruits and vegetables. Once isolated, the chemical compound was able to be reproduced and manufactured. Vitamins could now be made into supplements. In 1934, ascorbic acid, or vitamin C, became the first synthetic vitamin pill marketed to the public (American Chemical Society National Historic Chemical Landmarks, 2002).

In the United States, by the 1920s, the quest for supplementary nutrition was also underway. A biochemistry professor named Harry Steenbock was trying to solve a pressing problem afflicting poor children who lived in America's crowded cities during the Industrial Revolution. Widespread malnutrition in urban children had led to an explosion of rickets, a condition that softens the bones and eventually leads to malformation of the spine. At its peak in Boston and New York, it was estimated that 80% of children showed mild to severe symptoms of rickets (Holick, 2010). The cause was a severe deficiency in vitamin D, a vitamin that humans get primarily from the sun as well as from fish oils, liver, eggs, and certain mushrooms (Wagner & Greer, 2008). As families left the countryside and moved to the city, their diets became more limited, and their time was often spent in factories rather than in fields. This change had calamitous results for public health.

Dr. Steenbock solved this crisis by using UV rays to irradiate foodstuffs, infusing them with an extra dose of vitamin D. Irradiated milk became the key to combatting rickets, and within two decades the condition was virtually eradicated in America (Rajakumer et al., 2007). "Enhanced" foods quickly took off. Iron-fortified cereals, iodized salt, and pastas and breads fortified with folic acid were all common products in grocery stores by the 1950s. Today, many processed foods have been infused with some amount of additional vitamins and minerals (perhaps excessively so—but that is another story). Supplements and infused foods have changed the world: Some of the great physical hardships resulting from poverty and limited diet can be mitigated because of the discovery and synthetic reproduction of vitamins and other essential nutrients.

For example, vitamin A deficiencies are common in nearly half the countries of the world, leading to lowered immunity and sometimes blindness. This deficiency is the primary cause of child blindness (World Health Organization, 2018). In Guatemala, a pilot program was started in the 1970s to add vitamin A to a staple food, sugar. By the early 1990s, all major sugar producers in Guatemala were following suit, and infused sugar became the main source of vitamin A for the whole population (Dary & Mora, 2002). Experimental fortification programs such as this one are being tried in many parts of the world, holding out the promise of helping to end devastating nutritional deficiencies. Other examples of diseases associated with deficiencies include cretinism and iodine deficiency and fetal neural tube defects with folate deficiency in pregnant women. In both cases, supplementation of foodstuffs with these substances has become universal (iodine in table salt, folate in grains and cereals).

These are only a handful of historical cases out of many in which dietary supplements have had what amounts to a miraculous effect.

DIET: SOIL, NUTRITIONAL CONTENT, AND CONSUMER CHOICE

What is the role of dietary supplements for most of us today? Does the average American's diet have widespread nutritional deficiencies that might require the use of supplements?

On the one hand, the availability of a rich variety of fresh foods is certainly greater than it was a hundred years ago, and our increased knowledge of nutrition has in many cases prevented what once were common side effects of malnutrition. Great strides have been made in overall health and life expectancy since the early 1900s. But even in the industrialized West, where these gains are most dramatic, we now face new concerns about nutrition.

The problem has changed over time from a scarcity of nutritious food to simply a widespread preference for less nutritious food. Though a full discussion of the history of American eating habits is beyond the scope of this chapter, the recent research into what Americans eat and why shares the same undisputed storyline: The increase in processed and fast-food consumption in the U.S. has made it very easy for Americans to regularly eat too much salt, sugar, and fat and at the same time deprive themselves of necessary nutrients. According to the Centers for Disease Control and Prevention, vitamin D, iron, and vitamin B6 are the most common deficiencies among Americans. Among the demographics, some fascinating patterns emerge: Vitamin D deficiency affects only about 3% of whites, but it impacts 12% of Hispanics and 31% of Blacks. (Vitamin D findings are complex, however, and I will talk about vitamin D levels in more detail in chapter 7). Geographically, in the U.S., fruit and vegetable consumption is much higher on the coasts, while pockets of the Midwest and the South show the least healthy diets. On a different note, young women (20 to 29) have the lowest iodine levels of all the female age groups, which is highly problematic since iodine is so critical during pregnancy (Centers for Disease Control and Prevention, 2012).

These eating habits and their attendant health problems are widely visible and much talked about. But for those Americans who are doing their best to move away from a fast-food culture, another fear is deeply troubling because it is seemingly invisible: Is there a decline in the nutritional value of the foods we expect to be "healthy"? Even if we avoid processed foods, some worry that there is less nutritional value in the staple fruits, vegetables, and grains that we eat today than in the same foodstuffs fifty or a hundred years ago. Do we need to take dietary supplements to make up for what has been lost?

First, What Evidence Is There to Suggest That Food Itself May Be Less Nutritious Than It Once Was?

Several studies do seem to point to a drop in the nutritional content of common fruits and vegetables. In 2004, a study published in the *Journal of the American College of Nutrition* concluded there were "reliable declines" in the amounts of certain nutrients found in forty-three different crops. The study compared the United States Department of Agriculture nutrient content data for these foods from 1950 to another assessment of the same selection in 1999. Looking at thirteen different nutrients, the researchers found that seven remained the same, but six declined. The authors posited that changes in farming practices systematically worked to value high-yield crops over high nutrition (Davis et al., 2004; Davis, 2009). An often-cited study from 1997 conducted in the UK also found a decline in select nutrients. A sample of twenty fruits and vegetables compared the levels of certain nutrients between records taken in 1930 and subsequent tests performed in 1980. The study found multiple areas of decline. In vegetables, there was less calcium, magnesium, copper, and sodium; and in fruits, less magnesium, iron, copper, and potassium (Mayer, 1997). The author recommended more research to find the cause for this change.

Popular interpretations of comparative studies such as these have been quick to jump to conclusions and to spread their suspicions about what these declines mean. Environmental protection advocates Roddy Scheer and Doug Moss are often quoted in their confident assertion that "fruits and vegetables grown decades ago were much richer in vitamins and minerals than the varieties most of us get today." Why is this the case? They claim that the "main culprit in this disturbing nutritional trend is soil depletion: Modern intensive agricultural methods have stripped increasing amounts of nutrients from the soil in which the food we eat grows. Sadly, each successive generation of fast-growing, pest-resistant carrot is truly less good for you than the one before" (Earth Talk, 2011). Groups like the Organic Consumers Association insist that the way to reverse the effect of these declines is to purchase from local organic farms; they argue that pesticides, genetic engineering, and overuse of soil have led to costly nutritional losses. Many supplement sellers and health blogs have echoed this logic, lamenting the nutrients that have disappeared from the soil (Editors of *Delicious Living*, 2016). Could it be true that apples have lost 80% of their calcium since 1940 (Thomas, 2007)?

Others argue that these studies have been wholly misconstrued. Soil content fluctuates from field to field and season to season depending on a host of factors, making widespread generalizations across time very difficult. Comparing two samples from different years is not a reliable method to establish a long-term trend—nor do the studies themselves actually point to soil depletion as the cause behind the change. The Senior Scientific Advisor at Canada's Bureau for Nutritional Sciences, Robin Marles, writes that there is actually no hard evidence of soil depletion or of significant nutritional decline. Marles explains that what appear to be declines in these studies are well within the range of natural variation, the expected difference between the nutritional content from one apple to the next. He writes that "if soils were truly deficient, the plant would not grow well, resulting in stunted growth, low yields, susceptibility to disease, and malformed produce, so the farmer would not have a crop to sell." In other words, the extreme soil depletion argument is just bad science (Marles, 2017).

Still, Marles says that behind the myth of American soil depletion there is a small kernel of truth: In some cases, farmers choose crop strains that are bred for high yield, and these crops may show a drop in nutrient density. This is called the "dilution effect." The problem, then, may not be in the soil, but in the genetics of certain favored crop strains. Even when this is the case, however, Marles writes that the dilution effect is very slight and can be mitigated by fertilization techniques. It does not mean that there is a significant and widespread decline in the nutritional value of our fruits and vegetables.

This means that Americans who are eating their recommended daily servings need not fear that the potential invisible fiends of soil depletion or the dilution effect are stealing the nutrients out of their food. A 2015 United States Department of Agriculture (USDA) study supports this belief, finding that the average intake levels for "most vitamins and minerals were higher in 2000 than in 1909" (USDA, 2004).

The Preference Trap: How Do Our Food Choices (And Those of Our Ancestors) Affect Us?

Worries over soil depletion and nutrient density in crops focus on our food's inability to give us what we need. But perhaps what we should be most worried about is something that is largely within our own control: the kinds of food that we habitually choose to eat. Our food choices have far-reaching effects. Farmers and grocery stores respond to our choices by giving us more of what we want, whether or not that is what is best for us.

Jo Robinson, author of *Eating on the Wild Side*, argues that there *are* significant nutritional losses in our diets, not due to soil depletion but to human choices over time. Farmers have always valued and bred the varieties of crops that are the most pest resistant and high yield, and of course, that appeal to the tastes of those they are selling to. Sweet flavors win out over bitter ones, even though bitter vegetables are rich in antioxidants. These choices add up over time and have led to a situation where the foods that are most easily available to us are generally those varieties that offer us fewer nutrients.

Robinson writes that when the phytonutrient content of wild plants is compared to kindred grocery store varieties, the losses are "startling." For hundreds of years, farmers have been cultivating crop strains that are sweeter and starchier, but it is only now that we have the technology to easily see how dramatic the nutritional consequences of those choices are. Today, "most of the fresh corn in our supermarkets is extra-sweet," and "the sweetest varieties approach 40 percent sugar." This extra-sweet white corn was bred in the 1960s and became instantly popular. It has far less nutritional value than its ancestor, the dark, multi-colored corn harvested by American Indians for centuries. Today, multi-colored corn is almost never found in stores, except as fall-themed decor. Robinson claims that other crops have similar histories: "We've reduced the nutrients and increased the sugar and starch content of hundreds of other fruits and vegetables" (Robinson, 2013).

This leaves us in a fraught position: What is available to us and what is good for us don't always coincide. In the industrialized world, the major worry about food scarcity has almost disappeared, which has resulted in some wonderful improvements in the last one hundred years. According to a 2015 report by the United States Department of Health and Human Services (HHS), "Deficiencies of essential nutrients have dramatically decreased, many infectious diseases have been conquered, and the majority of the U.S. population can now anticipate a long and productive life." (HHS, 2015) Yet the effects of poor food choices still haunt us in an age of abundance: Chronic disease rates have increased, along with obesity. The Dietary Guidelines for Americans reports that, on average, Americans get more calories than they need each day but not always the recommended amount of nutrients (HHS, 2015). Educating ourselves about our food's nutritional value and going out of our way to find those varieties that offer us the vitamins and minerals we need is essential to bucking trends that keep us eating too much and getting too little. Diet will always be the primary way that our nutritional needs are met.

It is also important to remember that what we need from our diets changes over time. Men, women, different age groups, and those with special conditions have different needs. Women especially are likely to go through different nutritional stages. Iron is the most common deficiency all over the world, but in particular it affects women, who need more than twice as much iron as men do until they reach menopause.

Women also need more calcium over the course of their lives because they are more prone to osteoporosis, but according to recent data, we need to be cautious with over-supplementation of calcium because it may increase cardiovascular disease-related mortality (Jenkins et al., 2018). Pregnant and nursing women need increased levels of doco-sahexaenoic acid (DHA), iodine, calcium, folic acid, and vitamin D. Once adults are over fifty, both men and women need increased levels of calcium to combat bone loss as well as more of vitamins B6, B12, and D. Because older adults generally take more medications, they need to be very careful to make sure that their medications do not interact negatively with their dietary supplements (National Institute on Aging, 2015).

A person's nutritional needs fluctuate depending on his or her activity level, age, sex, and other special health considerations. Understanding these changing needs is extremely helpful in keeping our bodies well and is key to evaluating when supplements might be especially beneficial.

Another factor that should be included in the discussion of how our food choices affect us is the difference between organic and non-organic foods. In general, organically grown foods are less likely to contain pesticide residues than conventional foods. I will be brief on this topic since this book focuses on dietary supplements rather than organic foods, but based on my research and understanding, I believe that organic foods are safer and more nutritious (and they taste far better) than foods grown with pesticides. Although we do not have an abundance of scientific studies on the health benefits of organic foods, the current published studies report the positive impact of organic foods on human health. A recent French study that prospectively (a study of outcomes in a group of individuals over a relatively long period of time) investigated the association between organic food consumption and the risk of cancer in about 69,000 adults reported that a higher frequency of organic food consumption was associated with a reduced risk of cancer. The authors of this study suggested that further research is necessary to determine the underlying factors involved in this association. This does not mean, however, that if we do not have access to, or cannot afford, organic fruits and vegetables, we should avoid conventionally grown produce altogether. Fruits and vegetables are one of the best possible sources for essential vitamins and minerals, organic or not (Baudry et al., 2018).

DIETARY SUPPLEMENTS AND TRADITIONAL MEDICAL PRACTICES

Much of what we refer to today as dietary supplements are not vitamins, minerals, or other essential nutrients, but plants that may have medicinal value. These kinds of supplements have a very long history and include thousands of varieties of herbs that have been part of the practice of different traditional treatments all around the world. How should we approach and evaluate these plant-based supplements?

A few years ago, I did some field work in Tahiti, looking for Tahitian medicinal plants with potential anti-aging properties. While there, I was also able to spend some time with a Tahitian healer who was renowned for her skill in making herbal remedies. Halfway through my trip, even though there was more to see and do than I could possibly have time for, I had to put my research on pause because I was experiencing severe abdominal cramps. I knew from experience that the only thing that could help me was a high dose of ibuprofen, which somehow I had failed to pack when I was getting ready to come to the island of Moorea in Tahiti.

After experiencing a full day of cramps, I shared with my healer friend how much pain I was in. She went to her garden and carefully picked blossoms from her hibiscus tree. After examining each flower, she selected a few of them and boiled them in water, then let the concoction cool. She then gave me several bottles of this flower water and asked me to drink a cup every hour. I was touched by her kindness and did not want to hurt her feelings, so I thanked her for the remedy and started drinking it. In all honesty, however, I did not expect any relief. If 600 mg of ibuprofen barely helps with my cramps, how could flower water do anything? To my surprise, after the second cup, my pain became more tolerable, and after four cups it was gone completely. I convinced myself that this was a coincidence or just a placebo effect, and I stopped drinking the hibiscus water. The pain came back. Baffled, I started drinking the remedy again, and once more the pain was gone. My cramps continued for three days, and I kept playing the same game with myself. Finally, I had to accept that the hibiscus flower water was as potent as ibuprofen!

Humbled and convinced, I asked my healer friend if I could pick some hibiscus flowers from her garden and make more of the flower water for myself for future use. She smiled at me and told me that if I tried to copy her remedy it would not work because I did not know exactly which flowers to pick. She explained that they needed to be a particular shade of red and that the boiling time and temperature had to be exactly right to extract the pain-relieving properties from the flowers. This experience taught me the value of traditional medical practices using botanicals when practiced by experienced local healers. In the case of my healer friend, herbal remedy recipes had been handed down in her family for generations. Her mother, grandmother, and great-grandmother were all healers who were respected and almost revered by their community.

Around the world, traditional medical practices have recommended herbs and other natural ingredients, and not pharmaceuticals, to treat various diseases. Some of these natural remedies have worked for thousands of years and continue to be the first line of defense for many people in Asia and Africa. But in traditional medical practices at their best, the herbs and natural products often came from the healer's garden, not from a bottle. They are natural and not synthetic, and are given under the supervision of someone with immense skill and experience.

Many of today's botanical products are far removed from that ideal and promise more than they can credibly deliver. But it is true that some traditional medicines have stood the test of time and are rightfully drawing the attention of those who would like to avoid the potentially damaging side effects of some pharmaceuticals.

St. John's wort (*Hypericum perforatum*), for example, has been used since the time of the ancient Greeks to promote wound healing. Today it is often sold as an aid to combat depression. Scientific trials on the effectiveness of St. John's wort show mixed results, quite possibly because different potency levels of the plant extract are involved from trial to trial, as well as different levels and kinds of depression. There is some positive evidence, however, that St. John's wort can treat mild and moderate depression with the same level of effectiveness as some anti-depressant drugs. Although ongoing research seeks to identify the compound with potential anti-depressant activity, the current data suggest that several groups of active compounds within the plant may cause this effect. St. John's wort also has known drug-supplement interactions with common medications, such as some forms of birth control, antibiotics, and heart medications (NIH, 2016). The main mechanisms of action of these drug-supplement interactions are due to the fact that St. John's wort is a very effective inducer of several drug-metabolizing enzymes, which means that it causes drugs that are metabolized by these enzymes to be degraded faster, leaving the body with lower concentrations in the blood, which often results in lower efficacy of the drug. Used carefully, however, some patients can be relieved of their depression without the risks of prescription drugs (Jafari and Orenstein, 2015).

Black cohosh is another potentially efficacious herbal remedy. In recent years, due to published studies on the risks of hormone replacement therapy, women have been seeking out herbal remedies as a way to alleviate the symptoms of menopause. Black cohosh, a plant native to North America but often used in traditional Chinese medicine, is recommended to help with the hot flashes, insomnia, and irritability commonly experienced by women during pre-menopause and menopause. The active ingredient at work in black cohosh is unknown, but some trials nevertheless indicate that it is effective (Jafari and Orenstein, 2015).

Traditional healing practices and complementary medicine have had increasing popularity in the West. A National Health Statistics Report that analyzed data from 2012 showed that approximately 38% of adults and nearly 12% of children in the United States used some form of complementary medicine, spending nearly $12.8 billion annually, with average out-of-pocket expenditures around $368 per person (Nahin et al., 2016). Of all these practices, traditional Chinese medicine (TCM) is the best known and includes a variety of treatments and practices, from botanicals to tai chi and acupuncture. The appeal of such complementary medicine is twofold: First, it promises a more natural path to wellness than drugs; and, second, it approaches health with a holistic philosophy that seeks to bring the spirit and the body into harmony.

TCM supplements are derived from a wide variety of plants and animal parts. Many of these have been shown to be ineffective, and a few, like ma huang (also known as ephedra), can be fatal. But others live up to their long-standing reputations. In the 1970s and 1980s, artemisinin, extracted from *Artemisia annua*, also known as Chinese sweet wormwood, was rigorously tested for its anti-malarial properties. Today, this compound and its derivatives are the basis for malaria treatments all over the world (Fung and Linn, 2015). Several other notable TCM supplements are currently being tested in clinical trials. Danshen dripping pill, a popular TCM remedy that is composed of danshen (*Salviae miltiorrhizae*), sanqi (*Panax notoginseng*), and borneol, has been used to increase circulation and to manage cardiovascular diseases such as angina. A commercially developed mixture of this remedy (T89 from Tasyl Pharmaceutical Inc.) was investigated in an FDA-approved international and multi-site randomized clinical trial for its role in atherosclerosis prevention (U.S. National Library of Medicine, 2017). The results of this study showed that this botanical remedy can improve symptoms of angina (Sun et al., 2018). However, the vast majority of the thousands of traditional medicines used around the world have not yet been carefully studied for their efficacy or safety.

In the United States, herbs and plant-based remedies such as these fall into the same category as vitamins and minerals: They are classified as dietary supplements, even though they are used to help cure a disease or alleviate symptoms rather than to supplement the diet. This was one of the most significant changes made by the new definition of dietary supplements adopted by the FDA in 1994. It opened the way for these plant-based products to be sold as dietary supplements rather than medications that would require greater regulatory standards. In short, though traditional medicines are intended to promote healing and to work against disease, whatever we are buying in a bottle at a health store has two great shortcomings. First, it is unlikely that it comes directly from a healer's garden or is being used under the supervision of a skilled traditional healer; and, second, it has not undergone the scientific scrutiny to ensure the safety and efficacy that pharmaceuticals must go through. In the end, mass-marketed and unregulated herbal remedies sold as dietary supplements may be giving us the worst of both worlds.

CONCLUSION

Dietary supplements do have a place in modern medicine and nutrition. They can be powerful agents for wellness when used appropriately. Furthermore, traditional medical practices that recommend plant-based remedies and other natural ingredients have worked for thousands of years. I have no doubt that these remedies are effective if used in the right context, and I know that science is still in its infancy in its ability to understand their mechanisms of action and their possible interactions with pharmaceuticals and other supplements. We therefore need to appreciate that supplements have great potential but that much about them and their effects is unknown.

The critical questions that remain are these: *How do we know if we need a particular supplement, and if we do, how do we choose the very best supplements?* What do we need to know in order to avoid low-quality or contaminated products, and how can we navigate past potentially false advertising and find those companies that are trustworthy in their manufacturing? I will answer these questions in the upcoming chapters.

TAKEAWAYS

- Deficiencies in vitamin D, iron, and vitamin B6 are the most common among modern Americans.

- Our nutritional needs differ according to sex, age, and other conditions.

- Severe deficiencies may point to an underlying health problem.

- The primary source of our nutrition is our diet; supplements are not a way to compensate for poor food choices. Choose non-processed, nutrient-dense foods and limit fats, sugars, and salt.

- Avoid boundless optimism and total skepticism concerning herbal remedies; instead, check the science behind an herbal supplement to evaluate any risks or possible benefits. Be wary of synthetic versions of such products.

ADDITIONAL RESOURCES

- A snapshot of American eating habits and nutritional status: The Centers for Disease Control 2012 Nutrition Report.

  https://www.cdc.gov/nutritionreport/pdf/4page_%202nd%20nutrition%20report_508_032912.pdf

- Practical guidelines for choosing healthy eating habits: United States Department of Health and Human Services 2015–2020 Dietary Guidelines for Americans.

  https://health.gov/dietaryguidelines/2015/resources/2015-2020_Dietary_Guidelines.pdf

- An introduction to dietary supplements, federal regulations on the industry, and safety concerns: The Office of Dietary Supplements.

  https://ods.od.nih.gov/

- A survey of several herbal medicines and their safety and efficacy for women's health: *Women's Health and Wellness Across the Lifespan.* Jafari, M., and Orenstein, G. (2015). Women and Herbal Medicine. In Ellen Olshansky (ed.), *Women's Health and Wellness Across the Lifespan.* (chapter 5). Philadelphia: Wolters Kluwer Health.

REFERENCES

American Chemical Society National Historic Chemical Landmarks. (2002). *Albert Szent-Györgyi's discovery of vitamin C.* http://www.acs .org/content/acs/en/education/whatischemistry/landmarks /szentgyorgyi.html

Baudry J., Assmann, K.E., Touvier, M., et al. (2018). Association of frequency of organic food consumption with cancer risk: Findings from the Nutrinet-Santé prospective cohort study. *Journal of the American Medical Association: Internal Medicine, 178*(12), 1597–1606. https://jamanetwork.com/journals/jamainternalmedicine/article-abstract/2707948

Centers for Disease Control (2012, March 16). *CDC's second nutrition report: A comprehensive biochemical assessment of the nutrition status of the U.S. population.* https://www.cdc.gov/nutritionreport/pdf/4page_%202nd %20nutrition%20report_508_032912.pdf

Dary, O., and Mora, J.O. (2002). Food fortification to reduce vitamin A deficiency: International vitamin A consultative group recommendations. *The Journal of Nutrition, 132*, 2927–2933.

Davis, D.R., Epp, M.D., & Riordan, H.D. (2004). Changes in USDA food composition data for 43 garden crops, 1950 to 1999. *The Journal of the American College of Nutrition, 23*, 669–82.

Davis, D.R. (2009). Declining fruit and vegetable nutrient composition: What is the evidence? *HortScience, 44*, 15–19.

Earth Talk. (2011, April 27). *Dirt poor: Have fruits and vegetables become less nutritious?* Scientific American. Retrieved from: https://www .scientificamerican.com/article/soil-depletion-and-nutrition-loss/

Editors of *Delicious Living*. (2016). *The soil-supplement connection.* http:// deliciousliving.com/supplements/soil-supplement-connection

Fung, F.Y., & Linn, Y.C. (2015). Developing traditional Chinese medicine in the era of evidence-based medicine: Current evidences and challenges. *Evidence-Based Complementary and Alternative Medicine, 2015*, 1–9.

Holick, M.F. (2010). The vitamin D deficiency pandemic: A forgotten hormone important for health. *Public Health Reviews*, *32*, 267–283.

Jafari, M., & Orenstein, G. (2015). Women and herbal medicine. In E. Olshansky (ed.), *Women's health and wellness across the lifespan* (chapter 5). Wolters Kluwer Health.

Jenkins, D.J.A., Spence, J.D., Giovannucci, E.L., Kim, Y., Josse, R., Vieth, R., Blanco Mejia, S., Viguiliouk, E., Nishi, S., Sahye-Pudaruth, S., Paquette, M., Patel, D., Mitchell, S., Kavanagh, M., Tsirakis, T., Bachiri, L., Maran, A., Umatheva, N., McKay, T. & Sievenpiper, J.L. (2018). Supplemental vitamins and minerals for CVD prevention and treatment. *Journal of the American College of Cardiology*, *71*, 2570–2584.

Marles, R. (2017). Mineral nutrient composition of vegetables, fruits and grains: The context of reports of apparent historical declines. *Journal of Food Composition and Analysis*, *56*, 93–103.

Mayer, A. (1997). Historical changes in the mineral content of fruits and vegetables. *British Food Journal*, *99*, 207–211.

Nahin, R.L., Barnes, P.M., & Stussman, B.J. (2016). Expenditures on complementary health approaches: United States, 2012. *National Health Statistics Report*, *95*, 1–11.

National Institute on Aging. (2015). *Dietary supplements*. National Institutes of Health, National Institute on Aging. https://www.nia.nih.gov/health/dietary-supplements

National Institutes of Health. (2016). *Saint John's wort*. United States Department of Health and Human Services, National Institutes of Health: National Center for Complimentary and Integrative Health. https://nccih.nih.gov/health/stjohnswort/ataglance.htm

Rajakumar, K., Greenspan, S.L., Thomas S.B., & Holick, M.F. (2007). SOLAR ultraviolet radiation and vitamin D: A historical perspective. *American Journal of Public Health*, *97*, 1746–1754.

Robinson, J. (2013, May 25). Breeding the nutrition out of our food. *The New York Times*. https://www.nytimes.com/2013/05/26/opinion/sunday/breeding-the-nutrition-out-of-our-food.html

Semba, R.D. (2012). The discovery of the vitamins. *International Journal for Vitamin and Nutrition Research, 82*, 310–315.

Sun, H., Guo, Z., Li, L., Wu, N., Yan, K., & Yan, X. (2018) Confirmation phase III global clinical trial of a botanical drug in patients with chronic stable angina (CAESA): New treatment options for myocardial ischemia heart disease. J Am Coll Cardiol, *71* (11_ Supplement), A36

Thomas, D. (2007). The mineral depletion of foods available to us as a nation (1940–2002) – A review of the 6th edition of McCance and Widdowson. *Nutrition and Health, 19* (1–2), 21–55. https://doi.org/10 .1177/026010600701900205

U.S. National Library of Medicine. (2017). *Study of compound danshen dripping pills to treat acute mountain sickness.* National Institutes of Health, U.S. National Library of Medicine. https://clinicaltrials.gov/ct2 /show/NCT03270787

United States Department of Agriculture. (2004). *Nutrient content of the U.S. food supply, 1909–2000 (Center for Nutrition Policy and Promotion, Home Economics Research Report No. 56).* United States Department of Agriculture. https://www.fns.usda.gov/nutrient-content-us-food -supply-1909-2004-summary-report

United States Department of Health and Human Services. (2015). *2015–2020 dietary guidelines for Americans. 8th Edition.* U.S. Department of Health and Human Services. https://health.gov/dietaryguidelines /2015/resources/2015-2020_Dietary_Guidelines.pdf

Wagner, C.L., & Greer, F.R. (2008). Prevention of rickets and vitamin D deficiency in infants, children, and adolescents. *Pediatrics, 122*, 1142–1152.

World Health Organization. (2018). *Micronutrient deficiencies: Vitamin A deficiency.* World Health Organization. http://www.who.int/nutrition /topics/vad/en/

CHAPTER 3

WHAT'S IN THAT PILL?
IS YOUR DIETARY SUPPLEMENT SAFE?

STORY

Over my career, I have read many studies and reports on adulterated or contaminated supplements that have damaged people's health and sometimes led to fatal complications. When one of my friends was taking a "natural" weight-loss supplement and began experiencing severe heart problems, I suspected the presence of ephedra. In 2004, the FDA banned ephedra for exactly this reason: its high association with cases of heart problems. Sure enough, I was right. Though the product listed it nowhere on its ingredients label, her dietary supplement was illegally spiked with ephedra. In another instance, the daughter of a friend of mine started drinking valerian tea, a dietary supplement advertised as being able to alleviate symptoms of anxiety. Without knowing it, one evening she drank too many cups of that tea and became overly sedated, leading to a car accident.

I have also witnessed firsthand the dangerous side effects of drug interactions with dietary supplements. Twice I have seen friends admitted to the hospital with excessive bleeding because they were taking a blood thinner, warfarin (Coumadin®), at the same time as they were taking high doses of fish oil. And most recently, another friend almost went into liver failure because the "liver detoxification program" recommended by her naturopathic doctor elevated her liver enzymes twenty times above the normal limit. Luckily, her liver enzymes were tested one month into the "detoxification" program, and once she stopped taking the supplements, the enzyme levels started to decrease. If my friend had also been consuming alcohol, most likely she would have needed a liver transplant. Unfortunately, both professionally and personally, I have heard and seen far too many of these painful stories.

HOW SAFE IS YOUR DIETARY SUPPLEMENT?

Although there are many supplement manufacturers of great integrity that prioritize their buyers' safety and health, there are also those who are willing to go to outrageous lengths to deceptively sell dangerous products and make a quick buck at the expense of their customers' well-being.

The story of Dr. Pieter Cohen, a researcher at Harvard, is a chilling one. Concerned about the grave but often unknown risks of many supplements available on the market, he put together a research team to chemically analyze the contents of twenty-one different dietary supplements. The team was checking to see if any of them contained the ingredient BMPEA (beta-methylphenethylamine), which has properties very similar to an amphetamine and is not approved by the FDA for use in supplements (FDA, 2017). Dr. Cohen's team found that eleven of the twenty-one products tested did have BMPEA. He cautioned in the published report of his findings that this could be a threat to public health, and that this ingredient's safety should be rigorously tested before being available to consumers (Cohen et al., 2016). The FDA responded to this research by issuing public warnings to the companies at fault, demanding that their products be pulled from the market. Six of those products containing BMPEA were weight-loss aids sold by a company called Hi-Tech Pharmaceuticals.

Shortly thereafter, notice of a lawsuit appeared in Dr. Cohen's mail: Hi-Tech Pharmaceuticals was suing him for $200 million dollars because of the contents of his research. They claimed that their ingredients were safe and effective, and that Dr. Cohen's article and the

FDA's subsequent actions had cost their company millions of dollars. Dr. Cohen and his team were shocked.

Jared Wheat, the CEO of Hi-Tech Pharmaceuticals, had first thought of starting a supplement company while in prison on charges related to selling ecstasy. The news source *STAT* reports that in 2003, "The FDA forced his company to destroy supplements spiked with an unapproved erectile dysfunction drug. In 2006, the agency seized $3 million worth of his company's products containing ephedra, a banned and potentially dangerous stimulant." In addition, "Wheat and several Hi-Tech associates were arrested for running an illegal online pharmacy based out of Belize" (R. Robbins, 2017).

Dr. Cohen would eventually win the lawsuit brought against him by Hi-Tech Pharmaceuticals, but it was expensive, time-consuming, and frightening. Dr. Cohen believes that was exactly the point. In an industry where there is a lot of money to be made, suits like this are trying to bully researchers, scaring them away from asking the tough questions that could protect public health (R. Robbins, 2017). Even now, Wheat and his company are still at it: Hi-Tech Pharmaceuticals is in a massive legal battle over selling products containing DMAA (1,3-dimethylamylamine), an amphetamine-derivative stimulant that the FDA has not approved, while Wheat himself has been charged with money laundering and fraud (D. Robbins, 2017). Meanwhile, the company's products are still being widely sold. Despite all this history, one online retailer describes their products as setting "a higher standard of scientific excellence for the dietary supplement industry" and claims they produce nutraceuticals that are "unmatched in quality and efficacy" (Supplement Warehouse, 2019).

"All-Natural" Supplements Can Still Be Dangerous

In some cases, the greatest safety issue is a lack of knowledge: Not enough research has been conducted to know the wide range of effects that a natural substance may have on a human being. Many people associate the words "natural" and "organic" with safe—but remember that snake venom and poisonous mushrooms also meet those criteria! Only once a substance's properties and effects on human beings are well-researched can we know if it is safe and in what dosage it should be taken. Here are several examples of widely encountered supplements that can have serious side effects.

Guarana

Guarana is a popular additive found in many supplements and energy drinks that claim to "naturally" boost performance and energy levels. It comes from a little black seed that grows on a tree indigenous to South America, and it contains high concentrations of caffeine— much higher than the average coffee bean. In 2001, I diagnosed a colleague with guarana-induced premature ventricular contractions, or severe heart palpitations. She had been regularly taking a dietary supplement that had high guarana content. Her palpitations were so severe that she was scheduled to have a heart procedure. I suggested that she stop taking the supplement and then ask her cardiologist to re-evaluate her. After one week, she stopped having the palpitations. She was fortunate because she did not end up having a chronic issue. Had she continued taking guarana any longer, she could have faced serious heart damage.

Because of my colleague's case, in 2002, we published an article on this topic, "Cardiovascular Adverse Reactions Associated with Guarana." In 2010, *The Wall Street Journal* interviewed me for my comment on the safety of guarana. My message for the past two decades has stayed the same: Dietary supplements should be used with caution, and they should always be monitored. Guarana has not been extensively studied, and it will take more work to pinpoint the exact cause of the observed adverse reactions, but it's safe to say that consumers should approach such supplements with care (Baghkhani and Jafari, 2002). Even completely natural products can cause physical distress and harm.

Camu Camu

Camu camu, also from South America, has been labeled as an up-and-coming "superfood" (Coles, 2013) that has been reported to have high amounts of vitamin C and phenolic compounds (Langley et al., 2015). The wildly popular television personality Dr. Oz wrote that it "might just be our missing fountain of youth." Not only is it rich in antioxidants, but it may even be able to moderate and improve people's moods (Dr. Oz Show, 2014). However, just as with guarana, camu camu may result in heart palpitations in some individuals. There is no caffeine in camu camu, but it does raise serotonin levels, which can also lead to irregular and quickened heart beats. When camu camu is taken in excess, it can cause diarrhea and insomnia due to its high vitamin C content.

I personally observed this reaction to camu camu in a friend of mine during a dinner party. She had been taking the supplement for two days, and by evening of the second day she had developed a severe case of palpitation that made her light-headed and short of breath. Camu camu may have health benefits, but as yet, its risks are not well enough understood.

Ephedra

One of the most contested herbal supplements in the United States is ephedra. From the Chinese herb ma huang, ephedra is a stimulant. It was a popular active ingredient in weight-loss and athletic performance supplements until it became associated with heightened risk of heart attack, stroke, and incidence of death. Based on published studies, ephedra was associated with a significant increased risk (about 3.5-fold) of adverse effects such as psychiatric symptoms and heart palpitations. After investigating 16,000 adverse event reports and 155 deaths related to ephedra, in 2004 the FDA banned its use in dietary supplements (Harvard Medical School, 2004). Several dietary supplement companies appealed the FDA ruling, but the ban has remained in effect (Ronis et al., 2018). In 2004, adverse reactions to ephedra were responsible for 62% of herb-related reports to poison-control centers (Harvard Medical School, 2004). Since the ban, there has been a significant reduction in these reports. Researchers note that the "number of calls to poison centers related to ephedra poisonings peaked at 10,326 in 2002 and steadily declined to 180 by the end of 2013" (Zell-Kanter et al., 2015).

And yet, in spite of the FDA ruling to ban the use of ephedra, some dietary supplements on the market today still contain it, or other illegal stimulants such as DMAA, without listing it as an ingredient on their labels.

The Invisible Threats of Contamination and Adulteration

In many cases, we can guard against unintended side effects and toxicity by increasing our knowledge about particular supplements and their physiological impact on our bodies. The most insidious risk of taking any supplement, however, is adulteration. How do we know that a product's ingredients are true to the label, or that the supplements haven't been contaminated during manufacturing and packaging?

Contamination is a serious threat, and it is the major reason for FDA recalls of dietary supplements. Pharmaceuticals, steroids, illegal substances, heavy metals, toxins, mold, allergens—all kinds of unlisted substances might be present in a supplement due to fraud or neglect.

Products for weight loss, sexual health, and sports performance are among those most likely to have been contaminated and adulterated (Mathews, 2017; Outram & Stewart, 2015). A 2018 study in *Consumer Reports* examined protein powders sold on the U.S. market and found that "virtually all of the 134 products tested contained detectable levels of at least one heavy metal and 55 percent tested positive for BPA (bisphenol A)" (Hirsch, 2018).

The worst cases are those of outright fraud, or the adulteration of dietary supplements with synthetic drugs. A 2014 UK study on popular body building supplements found that sixteen out of twenty-four products that they tested contained anabolic steroids not listed on the ingredient labels (Abbate et al., 2015). Athletes may be shocked to test positive for steroids when taking these adulterated dietary supplements. One report noted that illegally adding synthetic drugs to dietary supplements often has an immediate payoff for unscrupulous producers. For weight loss especially, "Consumers tend to quit using those products if they don't realize any initial effects." However, "If the supplement quickly succeeds in providing the desired results, more units are likely to be sold, increasing the seller's profit." And so, "Appetite suppressors, stimulants, antidepressants, anxiolytics, diuretics and laxatives" are the most frequent adulterants found in weight-loss supplements. Without testing every weight-loss supplement on the market, it is impossible to say what percentage of these products are adulterated. But the chemical analyses that have investigated a handful of products at random are not encouraging. One research team looked at twenty-seven different dietary supplements that had been recalled at least six months before because of the presence of illegal substances but were still being sold. The analysis came back showing that "18 of those recalled supplements remained adulterated" (Rocha et al., 2016).

Sexual enhancement products are open to the same kind of abuse. For reasons related to privacy, cost, and the perceived ability to self-medicate through natural products, dietary supplements claiming to help with the problem of erectile dysfunction are a rapidly expanding market. Phosphodiesterase type 5 inhibitors (PDE-5 inhibitors) such as sildenafil (Viagra®) and its analogs are the most frequent adulterants. "Since 2010, FDA has issued 229 public notifications for sexual enhancement dietary supplements" that were spiked with PDE-5 inhibitors, comprising more than 55% of all the public notifications posted by the FDA about dietary supplements (Rocha et al., 2016). For men, unknowingly taking a PDE-5 inhibitor is risky and can increase the chances of suffering a heart attack. To make things worse, the generic formulations of PDE-5 that are used in adulterated supplements are often untested, of varying potency, and are much more dangerous than taking the FDA-approved formulations of erectile dysfunction drugs. These scandals tend to cycle: One company is exposed as a fraud and is censured or fined. But in the meantime, new manufacturers open their doors and start playing the same game (Sheridan, 2018).

The Bottom Line

The inconsistent quality and safety of dietary supplements come at a great cost to you and me. In the last twenty years, it is reported that "US poison-control centers have gotten about 275,000 reports—roughly one every 24 minutes—of people who reacted badly to supplements; a third of them were about herbal remedies" (Rao et al., 2017). In the same span of time, emergency room visits related to supplement use have risen "from 3.5 to 9.3 cases per 100,000 people, a 166% increase" (Brodin, 2017). U.S. Pharmacopeia reports that annually, 20,000 people end up in the emergency room due to supplements (U.S. Pharmacopeia, 2016).

We cannot assume that dietary supplements are safe because they are natural. Guarana, camu camu, and ephedra are natural products but are potentially unsafe for human beings. And even if they are safe in themselves, dietary supplements can be accidentally contaminated at some point during their manufacturing and packaging process. Unfortunately, especially in the realm of body building, weight loss, and sexual enhancement supplements, purposeful adulteration with synthetic drugs happens all too often.

Without denying the good that supplements can do, we need to be aware that the blanket assumption that supplements have no power to harm us leaves us unprotected from a dizzying array of negative side effects—some of which are life-endangering.

THE ANATOMY OF A DIETARY SUPPLEMENT

Now that we are aware of the risks of supplements, what are the steps for identifying a high-quality supplement? How can you make sure that you are not purchasing something harmful or fraudulent? How can you know if a supplement will work for you?

First, remember that dietary supplements are sold in many different forms. Some are a single compound, such as iron, but many are a combination of multiple ingredients. Most often, when we think of a dietary supplement, we picture a pill, but they also come as powders, teas, drinks, or gels. According to FDA guidelines, the criteria defining dietary supplements are that they contain a "dietary ingredient" and are intended to supplement the diet and enhance health. This broad definition means that tens of thousands of products can currently be in this category.

As a result, assessing the safety and efficacy of dietary supplements is like trying to ride a many-headed monster. To take even the simplest example, if your diet needs additional vitamin C, what kind of vitamin C supplement should you choose? Even if a product promises 200% of your daily intake, the formulation of that vitamin C product (tablet, capsule, liquid, etc.), along with the other nutrients present in your body, will affect your actual degree of absorption. The technical term for this is bioavailability. A quality product will effectively disintegrate and be absorbed by the average person, but a crude and low-quality formulation won't be fully absorbed. Some powder or liquid forms are more readily absorbed than pills, but they may also be more easily contaminated or spoiled. And, of course, the body can absorb only so much of a nutrient at once: A megadose of anything is likely to be mostly wasted, and in the best-case scenario end up in your urine or feces. In the worst case, too much could stay in the body and become toxic.

As an example, a shelf full of vitamin C supplements can offer radically different levels of bioavailability, even if their labels all appear to be very similar.

Reading the Label

To assess any supplement, the best place to start is to learn the language of its label as shown in the below example of a hypothetical label (Figure 1). FDA guidelines require that five key pieces of information be listed on every supplement label:

1. Statement of identity: the name of the dietary supplement must be clearly presented.

2. Net quantity of contents: the amount of the dietary supplement in each dose must be given.

3. Nutrition labeling: as with food, basic nutritional information is required.

4. Ingredient list: all the compounds in the supplement must be listed, along with any added "binders, colors, excipients, fillers, flavors, and sweeteners" (FDA, 2005).

5. Name and place of business of the manufacturer, packer, or distributor.

This is vital information. The label should clearly list the active ingredient(s), which is the substance that has a pharmacological or therapeutic effect, and their amounts (usually listed as international unit [IU], milligram [mg], or microgram [mcg]). It should also inform us about inactive ingredients (such as preservatives and fillers) and alert the consumer to any potential allergens.

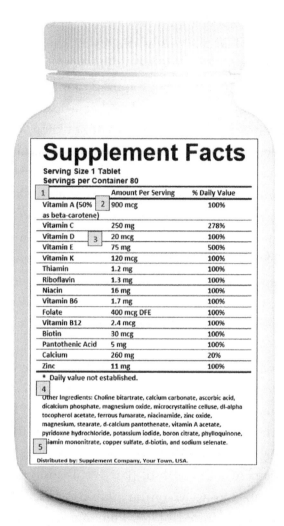

Supplement Facts

Serving Size 1 Tablet
Servings per Container 80

1	Amount Per Serving	% Daily Value
Vitamin A (50% [2] 900 mcg as beta-carotene)	900 mcg	100%
Vitamin C	250 mg	278%
Vitamin D [3]	20 mcg	100%
Vitamin E	75 mg	500%
Vitamin K	120 mcg	100%
Thiamin	1.2 mg	100%
Riboflavin	1.3 mg	100%
Niacin	16 mg	100%
Vitamin B6	1.7 mg	100%
Folate	400 mcg DFE	100%
Vitamin B12	2.4 mcg	100%
Biotin	30 mcg	100%
Pantothenic Acid	5 mg	100%
Calcium	260 mg	20%
Zinc	11 mg	100%

* Daily value not established.

[4] Other Ingredients: Choline bitartrate, calcium carbonate, ascorbic acid, dicalcium phosphate, magnesium oxide, microcrystalline celluse, dl-alpha tocopherol acetate, ferrous fumarate, niacinamide, zinc oxide, magnesium, stearate, d-calcium pantothenate, vitamin A acetate, pyridoxne hydrochloride, potassium iodide, boron citrate, phylloquinone, [5] iamin mononitrate, copper sulfate, d-biotin, and sodium selenate.

Distributed by: Supplement Company, Your Town, USA.

Figure 1. A Hypothetical Example of a Dietary Supplement Label

In addition to the above FDA-required information, the packaging of the dietary supplements often includes health benefit claims. Immediately after these claims, all supplements must print the disclaimer that whatever their product's health claims might be, the supplement and its effectiveness have not been approved by the FDA:

"This statement has not been evaluated by the FDA. This product is not intended to diagnose, treat, cure, or prevent any disease."

Though these labeling requirements are intended to safeguard and inform the public, the trustworthiness of these statements ultimately depends on the manufacturers. The FDA warns, "Under our regulations, label approval is not required to import or distribute a dietary supplement" (FDA, 2005). In other words, because there is no pre-market review or regulation, we cannot know for certain that dietary supplements contain what is on their label. What is more worrying is that, even if a product says that it is manufactured in the United States, this does not preclude the possibility that a U.S. manufacturer is buying its ingredients from foreign countries. A recent court case showed exactly that: DMAA, a chemical stimulant banned in the United States, was mixed in with the raw ingredients being sold by Chinese suppliers to U.S. manufacturers of sports supplements. In this case, the supplements' adulteration wasn't intended by the U.S. producers, but it happened nonetheless through their supply chain (Crosbie, 2017).

For this reason, investigating the manufacturer is perhaps the most important part of reading a dietary supplement label. A good place to start such an investigation is the FDA website (www.fda.gov), where you can search for the manufacturer's name to see if they have been investigated by the FDA. Other sources to check for the quality of dietary supplements are the third-party evaluation programs such as ConsumerLab.com (www.consumerlab.com), NSF International (www.nsf.org), and United States Pharmacopeia (www.usp.org) (Whybark, 2004). These programs do not systematically evaluate all the dietary supplements that are on the market. They often evaluate the accuracy of the label and the quality of the most popular ones on the market or the ones that they are invited to evaluate by their manufactures. In fact, in a study conducted by military treatment facilities, it was reported that of the 753 different products that were dispensed through 1.5 million dietary supplement prescriptions from 2007 through 2011, only about 3.6% of the products that were examined were evaluated by evaluation programs (Jones et al., 2015).

Behind the Label: Checking the Manufacturer

To check a dietary supplement's trustworthiness, look for those companies that have voluntarily submitted their products to be evaluated by independent regulatory agencies, which monitor product manufacturing and sales from start to finish. You may also consider checking the FDA website (www.fda.gov) to see if the FDA has sent the manufacturer any warning letters. Often, what is listed on the label is not what you would find in the supplement. In 2015, the New York State attorney general, Eric Schneiderman, led an investigation conducting tests on top-selling herbal supplements at four major retailers: GNC, Target, Walgreens, and Walmart (O'Connor, 2015). His investigation was prompted by a Canadian study that performed DNA barcoding on herbal supplements and found that 59% of the herbal supplements tested contained species of plants not listed on the label (Newmaster et al., 2013). Schneiderman found that four out of five herbal dietary supplements did not contain the herbs that were listed on the label. Ginseng pills contained only powdered garlic and rice. Ginkgo biloba contained radish, houseplants, and wheat. Some pills contained fillers such as peanuts and soybeans, which can cause severe allergies, without listing them in the list of ingredients. The attorney general sent the retailers cease-and-desist letters demanding an explanation of the process they use to verify the ingredients of their supplements. After receiving these letters, Walgreens, Walmart, and GNC said they would remove the fraudulent products from their shelves (O'Connor, 2015).

U.S. Pharmacopeia (USP, www.usp.org) is one of the country's largest and most credible independent regulatory agencies, investigating the quality and manufacturing processes of pharmaceuticals, food products, and dietary supplements. Many companies voluntarily seek out USP approval for their products, which requires them to undergo audits of their manufacturing practices, laboratory tests validating their ingredients' purity and potency, and ongoing spot-checking of the products after they are put on the market. This high level of quality assurance doesn't necessarily mean that the products are more expensive—many of Costco's supplement products are USP-approved! USP lists all its approved labels on its website, and the products that have passed their tests carry a USP seal.

NSF International (www.nsf.org) is another well-established and accredited independent board that certifies the quality of supplements and regulates businesses, especially those producing sports-related supplements. Consumer Lab (ConsumerLab.com) and LabDoor (LabDoor.com) are two more groups that regularly publish comparative reports on the top-selling dietary supplements. Their analysis is not as extensive as USP's, but they still produce useful reports. Another independent resource to check for information on dietary supplement safety is Natural Medicines (www.naturalmedicines.com).

Reading Your Body: Is This Supplement Safe for You?

Even when supplements are exactly what they claim to be—free of contaminants, easily absorbable, and in every way of the highest quality possible—*supplements can still be unsafe.*

Why? Because each person's body has different needs, stresses, and responses. In addition, each person may already be taking other dietary supplements or pharmaceuticals that could interact with this new supplement. Because of this, a supplement may be beneficial to one person and yet harmful under different conditions or for a different person.

My goal is not to create paranoia about your multivitamin or to scare you away from supplements entirely. But, if we take supplements seriously as agents for improving our health, we must be equally serious about the harm that can be done when we introduce a substance into our system that will create a physiological effect in our bodies. We would instantly recoil at the thought of a healthy person taking daily doses of cough syrup or blood pressure medication that they did not need, but excessive and unneeded doses of vitamins, potassium, or iron should also make us shudder.

In chapter 7, I discuss the process of evaluating your blood tests and discerning along with a healthcare provider whether or not there is a dietary supplement that would benefit you. If it is determined that a dietary supplement is needed, here are two more concerns that you should be aware of before taking a supplement.

Dietary Supplements Can Cause Adverse Reactions

Remember, every year over 20,000 emergency department visits in the United States are due to dietary supplement–induced adverse reactions. For young adults, the majority of these visits are caused by weight loss or energy products, while older people can have swallowing problems with vitamins, multivitamins, and minerals. Be mindful and on the alert for any problematic symptoms. For instance, if you are taking a weight-loss, energy enhancing, or body building product, you need to watch for cardiac symptoms such as palpitations, chest pain, or high blood pressure. According to a study funded by the HHS, weight-loss and energy products were implicated in almost 72% of all emergency room visits for supplement-related adverse events (Geller et al., 2015).

The whole purpose of taking a dietary supplement is to support your health, so you need to pay attention to how your supplement interacts with your body. For example, many supplements have trace amounts of gluten as part of their inactive ingredients, and while for most people this would be fine, someone with celiac disease should be very cautious about the fillers used in a supplement.

One of the most common adverse reactions caused by dietary supplements is liver toxicity. LiverTox® (https://livertox.nih.gov), a comprehensive database developed and run by the NIH, provides information on liver injuries caused by prescription and nonprescription medications, as well as dietary supplements. LiverTox also includes a case registry that houses all the published case reports on liver toxicities caused by drugs or dietary supplements.

Adverse reactions caused by dietary supplements are not limited to liver injuries. In a comprehensive review of the published studies on adverse effects of dietary supplements, it was reported that despite widespread consumption of dietary supplements by about 70% of Americans, there is limited evidence of their health benefits in well-nourished adults. However, some of these products—including some commonly used products such as fish oil, vitamins, botanical extracts, and protein powders—have the potential to produce significant toxicities (Ronis et al., 2018) such as increased cancer risk caused by β-carotene (ATBC Study, 1994) and spontaneous bleeding by ginkgo biloba (Bent et al., 2005).

Dietary Supplements Can Interact with Other Medications or Supplements That You Are Taking

Americans are prescribed an ever-increasing number of pharmaceutical medications. Roughly a third of adults taking those drugs are also taking one or more dietary supplements and are at great risk of dangerous supplement-drug interactions. This is a growing concern nationwide, and groups such as the National Center for Complementary and Integrative Health are pioneering research on these risky interactions (Hopp, 2015). But even so, it can take a long time for the public to become aware of and benefit from such research. Instead, individuals need to be proactive.

Before starting to take a supplement, you should ask yourself: Will this supplement interact with any medications or other supplements that I am taking? Ask your physician or pharmacist if it is safe to take a specific supplement in conjunction with your other medications and supplements. Also, if there is a significant change in your health, anything that you take should be re-evaluated. Someone undergoing chemotherapy, for instance, should not be taking extra doses of vitamin E or C, as some reports have argued (although not conclusively) that they might interfere with the chemotherapy treatment. Other herbal supplements, like St. John's wort, can diminish the effectiveness of birth control pills and antidepressants by speeding up the metabolism of these drugs (Office of Dietary Supplements, 2011; Ronis et al., 2018). Some of these supplement-drug interactions can be fatal by increasing bleeding. Fish oil and omega-3 fatty acids can promote bleeding in patients taking anticoagulant drugs such as warfarin (Gross et al., 2017; Buckley et al., 2004).

CONCLUSION

Dietary supplements can be helpful and sometimes even essential to our health. But they can be unsafe due to many factors: adverse effects, incorrect dosages, contamination or adulteration issues, and dangerous interactions with other medications or supplements. To ensure their safety, we need to ask the following questions before taking a dietary supplement:

- What is the recommended dose for this supplement? What is considered a toxic dose for this product?

- Does this supplement have any adverse effects? Are there any published reports on how these adverse effects may manifest in me?

- Is the supplement contaminated?

- Will the supplement interact with a medication or another supplement that I am taking?

- Who is the manufacturer of this supplement? Where do they manufacture their products? Where do their ingredients come from? Has the manufacturer received any warning letters from the FDA?

- Has the manufacturing process been reviewed by an independent evaluation program (e.g., U.S. Pharmacopeia)?

It is extremely hard to evaluate the quality of supplements, and nearly impossible for the average consumer to do so (unless they have access to a research lab). One of the resources for assessing supplement safety is independent regulatory boards and companies that test and approve the quality of pharmaceutical and dietary supplement manufacturing processes. The rigor of such agencies can protect consumers from false advertising and low-quality products.

And don't forget about your primary care physician, pharmacists, and other healthcare providers. Though many people fail to ask their healthcare providers about whether or not a supplement is safe and necessary, this should always be the first door that you knock on. The goal with supplement use is the same as with any medication or procedure: First do no harm!

TAKEAWAYS

- We cannot assume that dietary supplements are safe because they are natural. In many cases, not enough research has been conducted to know the wide range of effects that a natural substance may have on a human being.

- Most supplements on the market are never spot-checked by the FDA for quality control, and thus there could be a risk of contamination during the manufacturing and packaging processes.

- The adulteration of supplements with illegal drugs or other ingredients that are not listed on the label is also a risk and is especially common in the realm of body building, weight-loss, and sexual enhancement supplements. Thousands of emergency room visits each year are a testament to this problem!

- Some supplements have more bioavailability than others. The only way you would know this is if you have your own chemistry lab at home—or if you check the information provided by those who do! Use the links in the Resources listed below (such as the independent evaluation programs like U.S. Pharmacopeia) to check for those supplement manufacturers who have voluntarily submitted their products for testing (and avoid those that produce low-quality or harmful products).

- Even when supplements are exactly what they claim to be—free of contaminants, easily absorbable, and in every way of the highest quality possible—supplements can still be unsafe. Check chapter 7 on how to determine, along with your doctor, if you truly need a particular supplement.

ADDITIONAL RESOURCES

- Information on reported adverse reactions to the Food and Drug Administration (FDA)'s Center for Food Safety and Applied Nutrition (CFSAN) Adverse Events Reporting System (CAERS).

  https://www.fda.gov/food/compliance-enforcement-food

- Information on FDA requirements for labeling dietary supplements.

  https://www.fda.gov/Food/GuidanceRegulation/Guidan ceDocumentsRegulatoryInformation/DietarySupplements /ucm2006823.htm

- A list of USP-approved products and information on quality testing.

  http://www.usp.org

- Information on quality rankings of popular and commonly used supplement brands: LabDoor.

  https://labdoor.com/

- *Consumer Reports*' data on supplements and health.

  https://www.consumerreports.org/vitamins-supplements /vitamins-and-supplements-natural-health/

- Information on sports supplements specifically: NSF International product certification list.

  http://www.nsfsport.com/index.php

- Information on adverse hepatotoxic effects related to dietary supplement and liver injuries.

  https://livertox.nih.gov

- A database of potentially harmful dietary supplements: the NIH Dietary Supplement Label Database (DSLD).

  https://dsld.nlm.nih.gov/

- Operation Supplement Safety: A list of questions to screen your supplement for safety.

  https://www.opss.org/

REFERENCES

Abbate, V., Kicman, A.T., Evans-Brown, M., McVeigh, J., Cowan, D.A., Wilson, C., Coles, S.J., & Walker, C.J. (2015). Anabolic steroids detected in bodybuilding dietary supplements—A significant risk to public health. *Drug Testing and Analysis, 7*(7), 609–618. https://doi.org/10.1002/dta.1728.

Alpha-Tocopherol, Beta-Carotene Cancer Prevention Study Group. (1994, April 14). The effect of vitamin E and beta-carotene on the incidence of lung cancer and other cancers in male smokers. *N Engl J Med, 330*(15), 1029–35. doi: 10.1056/NEJM199404143301501. PMID: 8127329.

Baghkhani, L., & Jafari, M. (2002). Cardiovascular adverse reactions associated with guarana: Is there a causal effect? *Journal of Herbal Pharmacotherapy, 2*(1), 57–61. https://doi.org/10.1080/J157v02n01_08.

Bent, S., Goldberg, H., Padula, A., & Avins, A.L. (2005, July). Spontaneous bleeding associated with ginkgo biloba: A case report and systematic review of the literature. *J Gen Intern Med, 20*(7), 657–61. doi: 10.1111/j.1525-1497.2005.0121.x. PMID: 16050865; PMCID: PMC1490168.

Brodin, E. (2017). *The $37 billion supplement industry is barely regulated—And it's allowing dangerous products to slip through the cracks.* Business Insider. http://www.businessinsider.com/supplements-vitamins-bad-or-good-health-2017-8

Buckley, M.S., Goff, A.D., & Knapp, W.E. Fish oil interaction with warfarin. (2004, January). *Ann Pharmacother, 38*(1), 50–2. doi: 10.1345/aph.1D007. PMID: 14742793.

Cohen, P.A., Bloszies, C., Yee, C., & Gerona, R. (2016). An amphetamine isomer whose efficacy and safety in humans has never been studied, β-methylphenylethylamine (BMPEA), is found in multiple dietary supplements. *Drug Test Anal., 8*(3–4), 328–33. doi: 10.1002/dta.1793. Epub 2015 Apr 7. PMID: 25847603. https://pubmed.ncbi.nlm.nih.gov/25847603/

Coles, T. (2013). *Camu camu benefits: 11 things you need to know about the fruit.* Huffington Post. https://www.huffingtonpost.ca/2013/07/25/camu-camu-benefits-_n_3644392.html.

Crosbie, J. (2017, November 9). *Researchers just discovered untested, dangerous chemicals in several common supplements.* Men's Health. https://www.menshealth.com/nutrition/a19541981/nsf-supplements-toxicology-dangerous-preworkout-dmaa-ephedra/.

Dr. Oz Show. (2014). *Dr. Oz loves camu camu – And so should you!* The Oz Blog. Retrieved from https://healthygoods.com/blog/dr-oz-loves-camu-camu-so-should-you/

Food and Drug Administration. (2005, April). *A dietary supplement labeling guide.* Department of Health and Human Services, Food and Drug Administration. https://www.fda.gov/Food/GuidanceRegulation/GuidanceDocumentsRegulatoryInformation/DietarySupplements/ucm2006823.htm.

———. (2017, November 29). *BMPEA in Dietary Supplements.* Department of Health and Human Services, Food and Drug Administration. https://www.fda.gov/Food/DietarySupplements/ProductsIngredients/ucm443790.htm

Geller, A.I., Shehab, N., Weidle, N.J., Lovegrove, M.C., Wolpert, B.J., Timbo, B.B., Mozersky, R.P., & Budnitz, D.S. (2015). Emergency department visits for adverse events related to dietary supplements. *The New England Journal of Medicine, 373*(16), 1531–1540. https://www.nejm.org/doi/full/10.1056/NEJMsa1504267. https://doi.org/10.1056/NEJMsa1504267.

Gross, B.W., Gillio, M., Rinehart, C.D., Lynch, C.A., & Rogers, F.B. (2017, Jan/Feb). Omega-3 fatty acid supplementation and warfarin: A lethal combination in traumatic brain injury. *J Trauma Nurs, 24*(1), 15–18. doi: 10.1097/JTN.0000000000000256. PMID: 28033135

Harvard Medical School. (2004). *Why the FDA banned ephedra.* Harvard Health Publishing. https://www.health.harvard.edu/staying-healthy/ephedra-ban

Hirsch, J. (2018, March 12). *Arsenic, lead found in popular protein supplements.* Consumer Reports. https://www.consumerreports.org/dietary -supplements/heavy-metals-in-protein-supplements/

Hopp, C. (2015). Past and future research at National Center for Complementary and Integrative Health with respect to botanicals. *The Journal of the American Botanical Council, 107,* 44–51.

Jones, D.R., Kasper, K,B., & Deuster, P.A. (2015, July). Third-party evaluation: A review of dietary supplements dispensed by military treatment facilities from 2007 to 2011. *Mil Med, 180*(7), 737–41. doi: 10.7205/

Langley, P. C., Pergolizzi, J. V., Jr., Taylor, R., Jr., & Ridgway, C. (2015). Antioxidant and associated capacities of camu (*Myrciaria dubia*): A systematic review. *Journal of Alternative and Complementary Medicine, 21*(1), 8–14. https://doi.org/10.1089/acm.2014.0130

Mathews, N.M. (2017). Prohibited contaminants in dietary supplements. *Sports Health, 10,* 19–31. https://doi.org/10.1177 /1941738117727736

Newmaster, S.G., Grguric, M., Shanmughanandhan, D., et al. (2013). DNA barcoding detects contamination and substitution in North American herbal products. *BMC Med, 11,* 222. https://doi.org/10 .1186/1741-7015-11-222

O'Conner A. (2015, February 3). New York Attorney General targets supplements at major retailers. *The New York Times.* https://well .blogs.nytimes.com/2015/02/03/new-york-attorney-general-targets -supplements-at-major-retailers/

Office of Dietary Supplements. (2011). *Dietary supplements: What you need to know.* National Institutes of Health: Office of Dietary Supplements. https://ods.od.nih.gov/HealthInformation/DS _WhatYouNeedToKnow.aspx

Outram, S., & Stewart, B. (2015). Doping through supplement use: A review of the available empirical data. *International Journal of Sport Nutrition and Exercise Metabolism, 25*(1), 54–59. https://doi.org/10.1123 /ijsnem.2013-0174

Rao, N., Spiller, H.A., Hodges, N.L., et al. (2017). An increase in dietary supplement exposures reported to US poison control centers. *J. Med. Toxicol. 13*, 227–237. https://doi.org/10.1007/s13181-017-0623-7

Robbins, D. (2017, October 6). Atlanta dietary supplement mogul faces new criminal charges. *Atlanta Journal Constitution.* https://www.ajc.com /news/breaking-news/atlanta-dietary-supplement-mogul-faces-new -criminal-charges/GejzJKYfVLj0xUUFkzgEBN

Robbins, R. (2017, January 10). *A supplement maker tried to silence this Harvard doctor—And put academic freedom on trial.* STAT. https://www.statnews .com/2017/01/10/supplement-harvard-pieter-cohen/

Rocha, T., Amaral, J., Beatriz, M., & Oliveira, P.P. (2016). Adulteration of dietary supplements by the illegal addition of synthetic drugs: A review. *Comprehensive Reviews in Food Science and Food Safety, 15*(1), 43–62. https://doi.org/10.1111/1541-4337.12173

Ronis, M.J.J., Pedersen, K.B., & Watt, J. (2018). Adverse effects of nutraceuticals and dietary supplements. *Annual Review of Pharmacology and Toxicology, 58*(1), 583–601. https://www.annualreviews.org/doi/abs /10.1146/annurev-pharmtox-010617-052844. https://doi.org/10 .1146/annurev-pharmtox-010617-052844

Sheridan, K. (2018, April 5). *In "all-natural" sexual enhancement supplements, Viagra is often a hidden ingredient.* Newsweek. http://www.newsweek .com/2018/04/13/all-natural-sexual-enhancement-supplements -viagra-often-hidden-ingredient-873200.html

Supplement Warehouse. (2019). Hi-Tech Pharmaceuticals. https:// supplementwarehouse.com/collections/hi-tech-pharmaceuticals

U.S. Pharmacopeia. (2016, September 15). *Choosing a quality supplement.* U.S. Pharmacopeia. http://qualitymatters.usp.org/choosing-quality -supplements

Whybark, M.K. (2004). Third-party evaluation programs for the quality of dietary supplements. 64: 30–33. *American Botanical Council, 64,* 30–33. https://www.herbalgram.org/resources/herbalgram/issues /64/table-of-contents/article2752/

Zell-Kanter, M., Quigley, M., & Leikin, J.B. (2015). Correspondence: Reduction in ephedra poisonings after FDA ban. *The New England Journal of Medicine, 372*, 2172–2174. https://www.nejm.org/doi/10.1056/NEJMc1502505. https://doi.org/10.1056/NEJMc1502505

CHAPTER 4

THE SCIENCE OF DIETARY SUPPLEMENTS

STORY

About ten years ago, I was invited to give a talk titled "Clinical Studies on Popular Dietary Supplements." I accepted the invitation and planned to review classic supplements: multivitamins, creatine, ginkgo biloba, echinacea, vitamin C, fish oil, B vitamins, and glucosamine. I thought that I would have no problem finding enough high-quality randomized controlled trials (RCTs, discussed in more detail below), the gold standard of clinical research, to be able to present scientific evidence on the efficacy of these supplements. To my surprise, I was not able to find high-quality RCTs with positive results on the efficacy of most of the supplements that I was researching. I was shocked. How is it possible, I wondered, that so many people could believe that supplements were so good for their health, and yet the evidence of actual benefits could be so scant?

Of course, there were a few exceptions, one of which was a study on age-related eye diseases funded by the NIH. The study was robust. It included enough participants to be likely to be reliable. A research team conducted a randomized placebo-controlled trial that evaluated the impact of antioxidants and zinc on age-related macular degeneration (AMD) in almost five thousand patients. The study concluded that enough benefit was shown to recommend that people older than 55 with AMD should take antioxidants (vitamins C, E, and A) and zinc (Kassoff et al., 2001). As AMD is the leading cause of vision loss for those over fifty, this is a truly valuable finding. I was hoping to find stacks of clinical trials like this one, but ten years ago my talk ended up reporting mostly on how little research had been done on even the most commonly used supplements.

Fortunately, researchers are beginning to tackle this void. In September 2018, I was invited to present a talk at a workshop on "Enhancing Natural Product Clinical Trials," sponsored by the National Institutes of Health's ODS. One of the outcomes of this workshop was the publication of a manuscript that summarized what all of the participants presented and recommended in the *FASEB Journal* in 2020 (Sorkin et al., 2020). Efforts like these can contribute to a database of knowledge that can be used to inform the public health decision-making process and give us a solid foundation of information about what supplements really can and can't do.

RESEARCH CHALLENGES

Investigation of dietary supplements, especially supplements that come from botanicals (of which there are tens of thousands), are truly the Wild West of pharmacological research. Universal research paradigms and standards are being developed, but the process is fraught with difficulty because the territory is so new, the variables are so many, and the funding is so scarce. I know about these challenges firsthand since I do research on botanical extracts in animal models such as fruit flies. I will share a few of my own challenges with you in this chapter.

Inconsistency

Research efforts have thus far been plagued with inconsistency. The proper study of botanicals intended to treat specific conditions, for instance, requires the same precision as studying pharmaceuticals. Yet studies often are not able to be repeated by other researchers, or to be generalized, for a number of reasons, primarily because of the poor methodologies employed and failure to use standardized botanical extracts. The majority of these studies did not properly describe the ingredients tested: What parts of the plant were used? What were the growth, harvest, and preparation methods? How was the plant product processed and manufactured? How was the plant extract standardized? For a study to be useful, it must be clear whether the tested substance was an extract, a raw ingredient, or a finished product (Swanson, 2002). In a review of 81 RCTs that evaluated echinacea, garlic, saw palmetto, ginkgo, or St. John's wort, only 12 (15%) of these studies performed tests to quantify the content of the herbal remedy that was studied (Wolsko et al., 2005).

Too often, these essential details are missing or vary so widely from study to study that it is impossible to draw firm and reliable conclusions. I know personally how inconsistency can present a major challenge to research. I endeavor to test only high-quality botanical extracts in my research laboratory, and I always double-check their quality myself, even when the supplier's certificate of analysis for the botanical extract seems to be acceptable. Yet despite being very careful to work only with high-quality products, I have noticed that the harvest time and location can impact a botanical's quality, which may result in inconsistent outcomes. In 2006, my laboratory tested an extract of *Rhodiola rosea* on the lifespan of fruit flies, and we observed a 7% increase in lifespan. Two years later, I tested another extract of *Rhodiola rosea* from another supplier and we observed a 25% increase in lifespan. We analyzed and compared the extracts and realized that the second extract contained more biomarker molecules than the first one, even though both products had been approved with the same certificate of analysis and were ostensibly rated as having the same quality level.

Another challenge that leads to inconsistency in testing is regulatory issues. Each country has built its own classification system and corresponding regulation levels for dietary supplements, which means that the burden of proof for the supplements' effectiveness differs from place to place. Consider the common sleep aid melatonin. In the U.S., melatonin is sold as a dietary supplement; in Europe and Canada, it is not sold as an over-the-counter substance (Riemann et al., 2017). Or the case of the hormone DHEA, which in many countries is treated as a controlled substance, as it was in the U.S. from 1985–1994. But today the U.S. treats it as a dietary supplement that is available over the counter (Kornblut & Wilson, 2005). In fact, a dear friend of mine took an over-the-counter DHEA supplement, believing it would increase her energy, and she developed DHEA-induced hypertension that went undiagnosed for months. Her physicians ran a number of tests to figure out why an otherwise healthy young female had developed hypertension. I was also concerned and asked her to send me a list of all the medications and supplements she was taking. As soon as I saw DHEA on her list, I became suspicious. She stopped taking DHEA, and her hypertension eventually disappeared.

From country to country, there is great variation even when it comes to the most basic questions about dietary supplements, like recommended dosages and intended use. This poses a significant challenge to conducting research with universal reliability.

Bad "Science" and Overstretched Claims

But in its own way, perhaps the greatest challenge for good science is just overcoming the existing body of poorly done bad supplement "science."

And there is a lot of bad supplement science out there. *Natural Products INSIDER*, which provides information on sales trends to dietary supplement manufacturers, performed an online survey among their readers. The survey asked whether the company participates in clinical research, and if so, in what way. More than one hundred dietary supplement companies responded, and two-thirds of those respondents reported that their companies were funding and/or supporting such research. This, as *Natural Products INSIDER* wrote, seemed like very "good news" (Myers, 2015).

Upon further investigation, however, I realized that my definition of research is different from the way that most of these companies define it. For instance, testing the impact of a supplement with claims to enhance memory and cognition on only ten subjects in a non-controlled and observational study using memory tests that are not validated by the research community is *not* considered research—it is called marketing. Also, the results obtained from testing a dietary supplement in an *in vitro* cell culture experiment cannot be presented as a scientific study applicable to humans. As we have seen in the previous chapters, many companies have very little incentive to research their products' effectiveness and safety before putting them on the market, but they have every incentive to market and sell them with extraordinary health promises afterwards. This practice has led to a cultural oversaturation of bad science, especially online, where fairytales and outright fraud are pervasive.

This chapter will explore how to find what *is* scientifically known about supplements, explaining where to look for the most rigorous studies and how to evaluate their meaning. In the age of clickbait and targeted marketing, we will learn how to cut through the hype and avoid falling for misleading claims.

But first, we will put on our lab coats and (theoretically) do a little science ourselves. How do scientists test for supplements' safety and efficacy? What happens behind the scenes?

THE SCIENCE BEHIND DIETARY SUPPLEMENTS

I have written quite emphatically that most supplements require greater research before we should trust their claims. But what exactly does that entail? What kinds of tests should be performed, and how much can they tell us about what a supplement can or cannot do?

For instance, how can we prove whether docosahexaenoic acid (DHA), found in fish oil, can prevent Alzheimer's disease; whether coenzyme Q10 is able to lower blood pressure; or whether turmeric and curcumin, long used in traditional Ayurvedic medicine in India, can fight cancer? For those supplements that make condition-specific health claims, there is in fact a series of methods to scientifically test whether or not such claims are true. Or, if a substance's exact properties and effects are inconclusive, we can at least test for whether or not they are likely to do harm. I firmly believe that research on safety issues is as important as research on efficacy issues. In the following sections, I will describe various scientific experiments that are often used to make scientific claims. These studies vary from *in vitro* (in a test tube) to *in vivo* (animal studies) to clinical trials (human studies).

In Vitro Experiments: Studies Performed in an Artificial Environment Such as a Test Tube or a Petri Dish

The simplest, safest, and often the least expensive way to test the effect of any substance is *in vitro*: put it in a test tube, a flask, or a petri dish and evaluate it. Under a microscope and through other experiments, a scientist examines what happens when the substance encounters a tiny culture of cells that have been isolated from living organisms, such as humans, organs, microorganisms, or molecular entities such as enzymes and genes. These *in vitro* studies provide researchers with their first insights into a compound's efficacy, safety, and mechanisms of action.

As a trial run for supplements, these studies are essential, but a positive effect in a petri dish does not equate with definitive science, nor does it warrant recommendations for humans. *In vitro* studies only serve as a foundation for further studies: Based on the results of an *in vitro* study, scientists can ask if there is enough potential to consider the expense and risk involved in further trials on live subjects (study participants). Since what happens in an *in vitro* environment does not mirror what happens in an *in vivo* environment (that is, inside a living organism), the *in vitro* studies' results cannot be directly extrapolated to humans.

Why am I talking about *in vitro* studies here? Because significant and unwarranted health claims about dietary supplements are sometimes made based on *in vitro* studies. Curcumin (the active ingredient in the spice turmeric), for example, has been studied *in vitro* with specific types of cancer cells to great effect (Hatcher et al., 2008), but as we will see, these findings have not been as easily replicated in human studies.

It is important for us to understand that we cannot assume that an *in vitro* experiment's positive outcomes can be duplicated in a human body. As consumers, we need to remember that companies often leave out this critical piece of information as they try to sell us their products. Here, I will review just a few examples of unwarranted health claims promoted by businesses hoping to boost their bottom line. In these cases, manufacturers magically transformed the *in vitro* test results into solid "scientific evidence" for how their supplement would affect humans. Such small-scale exploratory studies, which might be a good beginning for scientists, are treated as the full story.

About a decade ago, marketers fell in love with the idea of antioxidants. Whether it was juices, cosmetics, supplements, or fortified snacks, many new products trumpeted their cleansing, antioxidant properties. For the first time, companies began advertising the "antioxidant levels" in their food products. The numbers were meant to impress consumers, and they certainly did: In 2011, sales of products advertising their antioxidant levels reached $65 million dollars (Berkeley Wellness, 2012). But what were these numbers representing? No *in vitro* measurement technique can tell us how much of the antioxidants in food are absorbed into our body and then remove potentially harmful oxidation products (free radicals) from our system. Whatever numbers we see on food packaging only reflects what happened in a test tube (and different tests seem to yield very different results). Yet, consumers' obvious assumption is that those numbers do reflect something meaningful about the actual health benefits of the products they are stamped on. The FDA chased down some of the worst offenders of overstretching antioxidant claims, including the manufacturers of Lipton Green Tea and Canada Dry Sparkling Green Tea Ginger Ale. Both companies received warning letters over their antioxidant claims and the purported corresponding health benefits that were used to market their products (FDA, 2010a; FDA, 2010b; Zajak, 2010).

Another hot product line seen by many as having health superpowers was the pomegranate juice product marketed by POM Wonderful, which was censured by the Federal Trade Commission (FTC) in 2010. The company's advertisements implied that its juices were able to prevent heart disease, prostate cancer, and even erectile dysfunction. When the FTC stepped in, the company was outraged, claiming to have spent more than $34 million in private research. After a fascinating court battle, the judge ruled that there was insufficient scientific evidence for the level of health claims being made. At the time, our local newspaper, the *Orange County Register*, called me to ask for a statement for an article that the paper was preparing about POM's health claims. The reporter asked my opinion about these claims and the science behind them. I told the reporter that people trust labels, especially health product labels, and that when companies are using scientific claims to sell a product, they should have scientific evidence to back it up (Hall, 2010).

One more intriguing example of the gap between marketing promises and scientific research is supplements that are derived from the spice turmeric. This golden root related to ginger was one of the top ten trending supplements of 2017, and indeed, the range of promises attached to it are spectacular. A CNN report published in 2018 goes down the list of enthralling claims: "Alzheimer's disease. Diabetes. Arthritis. Unwanted hair growth. Baldness. Infertility. Erectile dysfunction. Hangovers. Glaucoma. Cancer." If you have an ailment, there is a good chance that someone, somewhere, is studying whether turmeric can treat it. The report goes on to say that "there are more than 15,000 manuscripts published about curcumin, the active ingredient in turmeric, and about 50 manuscripts added to this collection each week" (Moulite, 2018).

How do we sort through the many studies and the barrage of speculation related to turmeric? Often, the first place that people turn to is a general internet search. If you look up "cancer and turmeric," for instance, the search will immediately yield a few dozen articles, blogs, and websites celebrating the discovery of a "natural cure for cancer." One turmeric website confidently touts the claim: "Research proves that turmeric and curcumin have natural anti-cancer, chemo-preventive, and radio-protective properties." The site proceeds to list many studies that seem to showcase why curcumin will revolutionize cancer care (Turmeric for Health, 2016). Of course, a closer look shows that the majority of the studies listed were conducted *in vitro*, outside of human beings, which we know means that they do not account for problems such as the limited bioavailability (absorption) of curcumin when ingested by humans. There is no way to guarantee similar results when curcumin is tested in a living organism versus a petri dish (Meyerowitz-Katz, 2017). So what can curcumin actually do? Internet summaries are not enough. We need to dig deeper and find the scientific studies themselves. And, out of all those studies, we need to look for human clinical trials if we want hard evidence of the effect curcumin (or any other supplement) is proven to have on the human body.

So what happens when curcumin is tested on human beings? A host of interesting findings emerge that highlight the complexity of supplement science.

Several human trials on curcumin's impact on colorectal cancer have been completed with conclusive results. Based on a recently published double-blind RTC funded by the NIH, there was no difference found in mean number or size of lower intestinal tract adenomas (polyps, which are the precursor to colon cancer) between groups of patients who received curcumin versus the group who took a placebo. When it comes to the development of colorectal cancer, the ultimate outcome of these intestinal adenomas, this clinical trial showed that curcumin had no effect in slowing or reversing its spread (Cruz-Correa et al., 2018).

On the other hand, clinical studies on curcumin's anti-inflammatory abilities have shown promising results in small-scale trials. In one of these trials, 367 people with knee osteoarthritis were divided into two groups, one taking ibuprofen and the other taking curcumin. After four weeks, the researchers concluded that on every scale of pain measurement, the curcumin supplements "were as efficacious as ibuprofen in pain reduction and functional improvement" (Daily et al., 2016). A related study on osteoarthritis tested curcumin's impact on biomarkers in the blood that indicate degeneration of collagen and inflammation. In an exploratory study, qualifying osteoarthritis patients were invited to take curcumin and then their blood was periodically tested to evaluate their biomarkers. There was no control group taking a placebo or other intervention to compare to those taking curcumin. The results were positive: Curcumin did seem to contribute to improved biomarkers. But the researchers were appropriately cautious because of the limitations of their research design. They concluded that the results were "encouraging" and a good indicator that more research should be done in this area (Henrotin et al., 2014).

Another recent human trial was conducted to test whether or not curcumin could improve memory, or slow memory loss, in aging adults. Though earlier trials in this area were inconclusive, this study, completed with forty middle-aged adults over an eighteen-month period, found that curcumin did improve memory and possibly also aided in brain health. The authors also openly acknowledge that Theracumin, a curcumin manufacturer, helped to fund the study, though there were many other supporters, from Alzheimer's disease organizations to the NIH (Small et al., 2018).

I personally have no doubt that curcumin has biological activities. I tested this compound in my laboratory and reported that it can increase fruit flies' lifespan and improve their healthspan by targeting longevity pathways. After the publication of my research in a peer-reviewed journal, I was approached by news media outlets asking me whether people should take curcumin in order to live longer. My answer was consistent with all the other answers I have given when asked this question about other natural products that I have worked with that have been shown to improve lifespan and healthspan: "If you are a fruit fly, curcumin can extend your lifespan." Of course, since we share about 75% of our disease genes with fruit flies, my hope is to eventually test my findings in mammalian model systems, such as mice, and ultimately humans. But as of now, I have not tested curcumin on mice or people—the jury is still out on whether it will lengthen human beings' lives or health spans.

So, what should we learn from all this? Curcumin shows many potential benefits when observed *in vitro*, but well-designed and replicable clinical studies are the only way to determine how curcumin affects (or fails to affect) a specific health concern. Each trial's design and size matter, giving us indicators of how much credence we should give to the results. Again, *in vitro* studies provide valuable information, but their main disadvantage is that it is often challenging to extrapolate their outcomes to humans. In the end, no matter what the internet's many voices are telling us, there is no surefire link between what happens in a petri dish and what will happen in the human body.

In Vivo Experiments: Studies Performed in Animals

Only through *in vivo* studies—those on living organisms—can it be determined how a whole living system, not just a small culture of cells, responds to the treatment. Many *in vivo* experiments are performed in so-called animal "model systems," including worms, insects such as fruit flies, and mammals like mice. Animal model studies are important and useful because researchers' overarching concern is to protect human beings from unintended negative effects; thus, efficacy and safety tests often do not begin with human populations but instead with animal models. But we need to keep in mind that animal models are simply "models": they are not humans.

In my own work, I conduct efficacy and safety tests on the insect model *Drosophila melanogaster*—better known as fruit flies. Since 2005, my research has focused on evaluating the impact of dietary supplements, including plant extracts, on lifespan and healthspan of fruit flies with the goal of eventually testing them in mammalian models. My lab has extensively studied five plant extracts that we identified after screening hundreds of compounds and natural products with potential properties to slow the aging process: *Rhodiola rosea*, *Rosa damascena*, curcumin, cinnamon, and *Angelica keiskei*. This process began with prior *in vitro* research and then graduated to whole system studies on fruit flies, which, as mentioned above, share about 75% of disease genes (i.e., genes whose function has been directly implicated in specific diseases) with humans. About half of their protein sequences have mammalian counterparts or homologues. We developed an algorithm to evaluate the impact of dietary supplements and botanical extracts on fruit fly lifespan and healthspan and then identify their mechanism of action. We are now in the process of testing their effect in mice before moving to human studies.

One of the common questions that I am asked about my findings from my fruit fly experiments (especially from the media) is, "Will this have the same effect on humans as it does on fruit flies?" (In particular, there was a lot of concern when we found that large doses of green tea extract harmed male fruit flies' reproductive systems!) I always provide the same answer: "If you are a fruit fly, this plant extract will have this impact. Beyond that, we don't know. Our findings need to be replicated in mammalian model systems and eventually humans." Lab tests on fruit flies provide us with a useful screening process; we can identify which plants may positively impact lifespan and healthspan or which plants may have negative side effects. Due to similarities between genes and proteins of fruit flies and mammals, we can also identify the potential mechanism of action of the extracts and compounds we are testing. But there is no way to extrapolate these results directly to humans without performing human testing.

Another commonly used *in vivo* model system to study dietary supplements is rodents. Mice and rats have played a critical role in biomedical research, from discovering drugs to testing dietary supplements. Although working with rodents is more expensive and labor-intensive than working with fruit flies, they are more convenient and less expensive than conducting studies on human beings. They have a shorter lifespan and can be housed and maintained easily, and their genetic, biological, and behavioral characteristics closely resemble those of humans. In addition, the use of "transgenic mice"—mice that have been manipulated to carry genes that are similar to those that cause human diseases—has created a new research platform to evaluate the efficacy and toxicity of drugs and dietary supplements.

In the case of both pharmaceuticals and dietary supplements, pre-clinical animal studies, using insects and mammals, that have sound methodologies are very useful for shedding light on the mechanism of action and screening for safety and efficacy. Often, after observing a positive effect in a study involving insects, the experiment is repeated in a rodent model, perhaps using mice. For instance, in my lab, after observing that a plant extract changed the microbiome (the microbiome is the community of all microorganisms that resides in living organisms) of fruit flies, we tested the impact of the same plant extract on the microbiome of a genetically engineered mouse model of obesity and diabetes (leptin-deficient mice) to see if the plant extract changed the microbiome of these mice. We observed that this plant extract did change the microbiome of these mice. Since the modulation of the microbiome appears to be conserved (in other words, to be maintained the same way) between two species, insects and mammals, we hypothesize that the plant extract may have the same effect on the microbiome of humans.

Animal studies may be useful in biomedical research, and it is fascinating to watch these studies evolve, but the bottom line is that they do not present a complete picture of whether or not the intervention will have preventive or therapeutic effects in humans.

Clinical Research and Clinical Trials: Studies Performed in Humans

According to the NIH, "Clinical research includes all research involving human participants. Clinical trials are clinical research studies involving human participants assigned to an intervention in which the study is designed to evaluate the effect(s) of the intervention on the participant and the effect being evaluated is a health-related biomedical or behavioral outcome" (http://www.nih.gov/). This broad description of NIH research reminds us that not all clinical studies have the same explanatory value; rather, there are many kinds of studies, each with different goals and levels of value.

Some clinical studies are observational: A researcher tracks what happens over time to a group of people. For instance, it has long been noted that people who eat Mediterranean diets have less heart disease (Hamblin, 2014). It also has been observed that India has a lower incidence of cancer than elsewhere. In observational studies like these, the observed fact is used as a springboard to theorize the cause but does not prove any cause conclusively. Could low cancer rates in India be explained by diet—turmeric, perhaps? Or do they have to do with a lack of detection? While cancer rates may appear low in India, a larger percentage of diagnosed cases are fatal, which may point to a problem with early-stage identification of cancers rather than a truly lower incidence of the disease (Dhillon, 2018). Observational studies identify interesting patterns, and we may speculate about their causes, but they do not provide us with a definite answer.

In addition to observational studies, there are other types of experimental clinical studies. For instance, a researcher may introduce a new factor and record the result. These experimental trials on humans provide us with different levels of evidence depending on their design, whether they are "controlled" or "uncontrolled." For example, if a group of people are all given a supplement said to improve mood, and are then asked after a fixed amount of time if their mood improved, they may all say yes. But how do we know that the weather didn't change for the better, lifting everyone's spirits? Or perhaps it was a placebo effect: people believe the pill will make them feel better and in turn do feel better. This hypothetical experiment may show us something important—perhaps the supplement does improve mood—but because the experiment does not control for the influence of other possible explanations (known as confounding factors) other than the effect of the pill, its value is limited.

The Gold Standard of Research: Randomized Clinical Trials (RCT)

The pinnacle of clinical trials on human beings is the RCT. These studies can yield the most meaningful data and are designed to prevent ambiguous and misleading outcomes. In an RCT, at least two groups of participants are necessary, one of which is given a placebo (the control), while the other is given the substance being studied (the intervention). In a "blinded" study, the participants don't know which group they are in. In a so-called "double-blinded" study, the researchers evaluating the outcomes of the study also don't know which group a patient is in until the results are finalized. The study participants need to be matched for all relevant characteristics (e.g., sex, age, race/ethnicity, other medical conditions) and are then randomized to either the control or the intervention group. The control group is the standard by which the researcher measures the effect of the intervention. The researchers measure and record the impact of control and intervention on outcomes that were hypothesized beforehand. After a given period, the researcher stops the experiment and analyzes the data. They may replicate the experiments to assure that their results are valid. The design of an RCT eliminates the possible interference of a placebo effect and controls for external and confounding factors that might skew the results.

What does a well-designed RCT look like, and what kinds of things can we learn from them?

One landmark RCT was conducted in 2005 on the long-term

effects of vitamin E supplementation on heart problems. In a seven-year study, a Canadian research team followed nearly 10,000 adults over 55 who were considered at high risk for heart attack or stroke. Half of the participants were given high doses of vitamin E every day, and the other half took a placebo pill. After seven years, there was no reduction in heart attacks, stroke, or cancer for the group taking vitamin E. There was, however, a 13% *increased* risk of heart failure in the group taking vitamin E (Lonn et al., 2005). Other studies have had similar results. In a study that evaluated the impact of selenium and vitamin E for cancer prevention, researchers found an increased incidence of prostate cancer in healthy men consuming these supplements (Klein et al., 2011). Despite the promising *in vitro*, animal, and observational studies on vitamin E, clinical trials in humans show no benefits and actually some risk (Vivekananthan et al., 2003).

In 2018, another significant study was published on the impact of dietary supplements on heart disease. Multiple researchers worked together to compile and analyze the results of over one thousand RCTs completed between 2012 and 2017. The RCTs included in this compilation, known as a "meta-analysis," were all testing for a relationship between particular supplements and the prevention of cardiovascular disease. The results of their meta-analysis are fascinating: First, there was no discernable effect on cardiovascular health found in the trial populations taking multivitamins, vitamins C or D, beta-carotene, calcium, or selenium. There was, however, some evidence of preventive benefits for the heart health of those who took folic acid, and fewer incidences of stroke for those who took B vitamins. Finally, there was increased risk for overall mortality found in studies of those taking antioxidant mixtures and niacin. Even with such an overwhelming wealth of studies to draw from, the authors acknowledge that much remains unknown. Depending on an individual's age, health, and dietary background, the benefits or potential dangers of taking any supplement will vary (Jenkins al., 2018).

Studies like this one are a good place to start. Such studies provide us with the best summary of what is presently known about supplements and what they can and cannot do.

A GRAIN OF SALT: YOUNG SCIENCE, OLD EARTH

Ideally, every supplement and its health claims would go through the appropriate progression of scientific studies, establishing if there is any benefit or risk, and what the level of efficacy is. But, of course, this process is rarely so clean-cut. In the case of botanicals, only a fraction of the properties of the hundreds of thousands of plants that exist have been tested for. For vitamins and minerals, an important part of future testing, in addition to efficacy, is to establish safety and dosage limits. We largely know what deficiency looks like for essential vitamins and minerals, but in cases where additional vitamin doses are theorized to help with specific health problems, there is still much left to learn. In relation to supplements and their potential, the science is still very young.

Having said that, as I stated in chapter 2, although scientific certainty is the goal, some traditional medical practices that have worked for thousands of years are likely to continue working if practiced in the right context, science or no science.

CHOOSING SUPPLEMENTS WISELY

Unlike pharmaceuticals, the major driver behind supplement use is personal choice rather than a prescription from a physician. Most people who are using supplements do so based on their own research, faith in advertising claims, or others' recommendations. Very few people are aware of the results of human RCTs like the ones discussed above. Instead, anecdotes ("My friend's sister started taking this and now her skin is perfect!") and endorsements are key motivators and clues that point people toward products. As we will see in the next chapter, celebri-docs like Dr. Oz can create instant "new" fads each time they air, spiking sales of hitherto little-heard-of supplements overnight (Woolston, 2012). But these anecdotes, whether from friends, celebrities, or personal testimonies found on blogs, are *not* science.

Even what appear to be scientific studies are not always trust-worthy: sources matter. Because supplement manufacturers can only make very limited claims on their products' packaging or they will be in trouble with the FTC or the FDA, websites and social media outlets are the perfect place to informally drum up enthusiasm for their products. Marketing and self-promotion are often presented as "research" and "science."

Studies can also be purposely designed with bias, guaranteeing that companies or individuals get the results they want, rather than presenting the full picture. This is easy to see in the growing market for weight-loss supplements. Each and every company hustling to sell their natural weight-loss aid will tell consumers that there is scientific evidence that their weight-loss supplement works (and, no doubt, will flash dramatic before-and-after pictures to prove it).

But science tells another story. One research team reviewed the results of nine different sets of clinical trials on human beings, all of which sought to test whether or not a given dietary supplement could help with weight loss. Each of the experiments lasted for at least twelve weeks, and they covered a wide range of dietary supplements: guar gum, chromium, ephedra, *Citrus aurantium*, conjugated linoleic acid, calcium, glucomannan, chitosan, and green tea. What was the conclusion? Based on the studies' results and quality, the reviewers wrote that these clinical trials "fail to provide good evidence that any of these preparations generate clinically relevant weight loss without undue risks" (Pittler and Ernst, 2004).

The fine print revealed that several of the supplements, such as chromium, might show potential for a very small increase in weight loss, but that the trials conducted thus far were not robust enough to be considered strong evidence. Ephedra was the only one that truly showed a significant effect on weight loss, but the serious risks, such as heart disease, of taking ephedra are also well known. Based on this review, there are no safe and effective weight-loss supplements on the market, and most of the studies that claim otherwise are poorly constructed and untrustworthy (Pittler and Ernst, 2004).

In addition, even well-designed studies may be cherry-picked or abused; numbers do not simply speak for themselves. You don't have to be a science professor to know that any kind of data can easily be manipulated. Interpreting the meaning of quantitative results is the art of good science, but all too often, misconstruing data is part of effective (if immoral) marketing campaigns. A good scientific publication presents its findings but also states the study's limitations and encourages the reader to do their homework prior to extrapolating these findings to their own life. A good scientific study will also inform the reader about who funded the study and if the authors and investigators had any potential conflict of interest with the supplement's manufacturer. An analysis of the press releases and news stories that were generated in response to clinical studies of dietary supplements revealed that 100% of the industry press releases hyped results or de-emphasized negative findings compared to 55% of the non-industry press releases. The authors concluded that the press releases of the dietary supplement industry emphasize results that are favorable to supplement use and downplay results that are not (Wang et al., 2014).

WHERE TO FIND GOOD SCIENCE ON DIETARY SUPPLEMENTS

So where should we look for the scientific studies on supplements, and how can we read them well?

Studies that showcase true scientific research will show up in professional and peer-reviewed journals, which means that other experts in the field reviewed the data's quality before the study was published. Fortunately, independent organizations like U.S. Pharmacopeia and federal research institutions like the NIH's ODS provide user-friendly compendiums of the latest research on supplements. The goal is to link the public to the scientific community, making the best research available to all. Having said that, not all the studies that have been published in scientific peer-reviewed journals are solid and can be replicated. A survey of 1,576 scientists conducted by one of the most prestigious scientific journals, *Nature*, reported, "70% of researchers have tried and failed to reproduce another scientist's experiments, and more than half have failed to reproduce their own experiments" (Baker, 2016). I have personally failed to reproduce the results of natural product studies published by others. If I fail to reproduce the results of my own experiments, then I present the data as negative unless additional replications (at least two more positive studies) point to the contrary. The National Institutes of Health recently developed guidelines to address so-called "rigor and reproducibility" in NIH-funded studies. Future surveys and studies that attempt to reproduce experiments will test the impact that these guidelines might have on the quality of scientific studies. Science-based medicine has improved human health over the last 150 years, and I certainly believe that it will continue to do so.

Despite concerns regarding reproducibility of studies on drugs and dietary supplements, here are the places to find the very best science on supplements:

National Institutes of Health's Office of Dietary Supplements Evidence-Based Review Program

Since 2001, the NIH ODS (ODS, 2001) has been part of a large-scale project to review the existing scientific studies related to supplements and to create recommendations for further areas of investigation. Draining one little corner of the swamp at a time, they are encouraging the science behind supplements to catch up to their claims (and sales!). Through the ODS Evidence-Based Review Program, peer-reviewed journal articles that examine the effects of vitamin D, soy, B vitamins, omega-3 fatty acids, multivitamins, and several other common supplements are made accessible to the public.

Information on various dietary supplements may be found at http://www.ods.od.nih.gov/.

In September 2018, I presented in a workshop organized by ODS titled "Enhancing Natural Product Clinical Trials." The workshop's goal was to develop and publicize good practices for various stages of research on natural products, including dietary supplements, from *in vitro* assays to clinical trials. Concentrated efforts such as this by the NIH are a significant step toward assuring the quality of research and publications on dietary supplements.

National Institute of Health Consortium for Advancing Research on Botanical and Other Natural Products (CARBON) Program

The CARBON program was initiated by the NIH ODS to promote collaborative research on efficacy, safety, and mechanism of action of botanical dietary supplements with high potential to benefit human health. Other centers and institutes at NIH, such as National Center for Complimentary and Integrative Health and National Institute on Aging (NIA), collaborate with this program and award funding to research centers and academic institutions with the goal of advancing research on botanical dietary supplements.

National Institutes of Health Clinical Trials

Anyone can find out if a supplement's efficacy and safety has ever been systematically tested on humans. All clinical trials on human beings, whether publicly or privately funded, must be approved by institutional review boards at each research institution, and every study is then registered with the federal government. Fortunately, these studies are available to the public through a federal website, www.clinicaltrials.gov/. However, we need to remember that just because a clinical trial is listed on this website, it does not mean that the clinical study is high quality. In the next section of this chapter, I will give you some basic questions to ask when assessing clinical studies.

The Food and Drug Administration

Another way to learn whether a product's health claims have any basis is to search the FDA catalog of investigations. If the FDA sent a letter of injunction or seizure concerning a supplement, often it is because a company was caught making a false scientific claim or the product was harming the public. By typing the name of the company in the search box of www.fda.gov/, anyone can access warning letters that the FDA has sent to that company. We need to remember that in most cases, by the time FDA starts investigating a company, that company's products have already harmed the public.

GOOD QUESTIONS TO ASK

We need to remember again that only the results of clinical studies can be extrapolated to humans. *In vitro* and animal studies are useful, but their results do not transfer into prescriptions for human health.

Without having to become an expert in research methodologies, consumers can still look for several key markers in clinical studies to interpret a particular study's meaning. Here are the questions that you should ask:

1. First, research methodology is important. How many participants were there? Was this a small study of a hundred people or less? Or was it a large study? The study's size and length can help us see whether it was exploratory in nature or if the findings are well-established. Was the study controlled, randomized, and blinded (that is, the patients or subjects don't know what treatment they're receiving)? It is important that the dietary supplement being tested is compared to a placebo or an established intervention in a randomized and blinded manner. If not, the significance of the study's findings is greatly diminished.

2. Next, where did the funding come from? Sound research can of course come from private sources, but we should be extra careful if a supplement manufacturer or another party financially vested in the outcome is funding the project. As we saw in chapter 1, the funding for research on the effectiveness of dietary supplements is sparse overall. The NIH and ODS are the primary sources of federal research dollars on dietary supplements, but many independent foundations also fund research on dietary supplements. The source of funding for the study should appear in the paper under the acknowledgements section.

3. Finally, where was the study published? Was it in a peer-reviewed journal, where reviewers had access to the primary data underlying the study? Or was it published in a newsletter, online blog, or website that is sponsored directly or indirectly by the dietary supplement manufacturer?

CONCLUSION

The science behind dietary supplements is still young, working against a tidal wave of conjecture. We must be careful about so-called scientific claims and adopt the mentality of a skeptical investigator as we approach supplements. High-quality companies should be more than happy to publish and share their research findings with you so that you can see for yourself how their study was conducted and find out the source of support for that study. Spending some time on finding answers to the questions that were presented above may not only save you a lot of money, but can also ensure the efficacy and safety of the supplement you are taking. After all, we all need to learn to make informed decisions about our health.

TAKEAWAYS

- There is a significant lack of research on the efficacy and safety of most dietary supplements.

- Much of the research that has been done is inconsistent, lacks standardization, and is not easily replicated. Another hurdle is that dietary supplements are legally categorized and treated differently from country to country.

- Perhaps the greatest problem is that there is a profusion of "bad" science concerning supplements: overstretched claims, biased studies designed to promote a product, and marketing materials that are packaged and presented as if they were scientific research (but aren't!).

- The key to understanding real scientific studies and what they mean is to be familiar with the types of studies that can be conducted on dietary supplements, and what we can learn from each level of study.

In Vitro: Studies performed in an artificial environment such as a test tube

In Vivo: Studies performed on live subjects such as animals

Clinical Research: Studies performed on human beings

- We cannot extrapolate results from one level of study to the next: What happens in a test tube is not guaranteed to happen in a human body! If an *in vitro* study shows that a substance fights cancer cells in a petri dish, we *cannot* take that as proof that the same substance will fight cancer in a human body.

- Different studies are designed for different purposes. Some are observational, while others are experimental. Some are controlled and others are uncontrolled. The study's design and size (and whether or not it has been replicated) can tell us how much validity the results of that study have.

- Before buying a product, look for whether that product has been the subject of an RCT. These are the most trustworthy of studies and can tell us about a supplement's safety and efficacy on humans over time.

- All clinical trials performed on human beings in the United States are reported to the federal government, which lists them all on this website: www.clinicaltrials.gov.

- When looking at a study, check to see whether it was a small or large study, was controlled (measures are taken to remove outside factors that could skew the results) or uncontrolled, and was randomized and blinded. Look to see where the funding came from (hopefully not from Buy More Supplements, Inc.). Check to see where it was published. Was it credible enough to be in a peer-reviewed journal?

ADDITIONAL RESOURCES

- Research resources on dietary supplements.

  Food and Drug Administration (www.FDA.gov)

  National Institute of Health's Clinical Trials (clinicaltrials.gov)

  NIH's Office of Dietary Supplements: Evidence-Based Review Program

  (https://ods.od.nih.gov/Research/Evidence-Based_Review_Program.aspx)

- Information on how to read and interpret scientific studies:

  "Dietary Supplements: A Framework for Evaluating Safety," produced by the Institute of Medicine and National Research Council.

  (https://www.nap.edu/catalog/10882/dietary-supplements-a-framework-for-evaluating-safety)

  "Randomised Controlled Trials—the gold standard for effectiveness research"

  https://www.ncbi.nlm.nih.gov/pmc/articles/PMC6235704/

REFERENCES

Baker, M. (2016). Is there a reproducibility crisis? A Nature survey lifts the lid on how researchers view the "crisis" rocking science and what they think will help. *Nature, 533*(7604), 452–454. https://www.nature .com/news/1-500-scientists-lift-the-lid-on-reproducibility-1.19970

Berkeley Wellness. (2012). *Beware of antioxidant claims.* University of California: Berkeley Wellness. http://www.berkeleywellness.com /healthy-eating/nutrition/article/beware-antioxidant-claims

Cruz-Correa, M., Hylind, L.M., Marrero, J.H., Zahurak, M.L., Murray-Stewart, T., Casero, R.A., Montgomery, E.A., et al. (2018). Efficacy and safety of curcumin in treatment of intestinal adenomas in patients with familial adenomatous polyposis. *Gastroenterology, 155*(3), 668.

Daily, J.W., Yang, M., & Park, S. (2016). Efficacy of turmeric extracts and curcumin for alleviating the symptoms of joint arthritis: A systematic review and meta-analysis of randomized clinical trials. *Journal of Medicinal Food, 19*(8), 717–29.

Dhillon, D. (2018). *No, India's rate of cancer incidence isn't among the lowest in the world.* Business Insider: India. https://www.businessinsider.in/no -indias-rate-of-cancer-incidence-isnt-among-the-lowest-in-the-world /articleshow/64464471.cms

Food and Drug Administration. (2010a, August 23). *Inspections, compliance, enforcement, and criminal investigations.* Department of Health and Human Services, Food and Drug Administration. https://wayback .archive-it.org/7993/20170112194422/http:/www.fda.gov/ICECI /EnforcementActions/WarningLetters/2010/ucm224509.htm

———. (2010b, August 30). *Inspections, compliance, enforcement, and criminal investigations.* Department of Health and Human Services, Food and Drug Administration. https://wayback.archive-it.org/7993 /20170112194410/http:/www.fda.gov/ICECI/EnforcementActions /WarningLetters/2010/ucm224571.htm

Hall, L. (2010, September 28). Are the feds really persecuting the pomegranate? *Orange County Register*. https://www.ocregister.com/2010/09/28/are-the-feds-really-persecuting-the-pomegranate/

Hamblin, J. (2014, March 24). *Science compared every diet, and the winner is real food*. The Atlantic. https://www.theatlantic.com/health/archive/2014/03/science-compared-every-diet-and-the-winner-is-real-food/284595/

Hatcher, H., Planalp, R., Cho, J., Torti, F.M., & Torti, S.V. (2008). Curcumin: From ancient medicine to current clinical trials. *Cellular and Molecular Life Sciences, 65*(11), 1631–52.

Henrotin, Y.E., Gharbi, M., Dierckxsens, Y., Priem, F., Marty, M., Seidel, L., Albert, A.I., Heuse, E., Bonnet, V., & Castermans, C. (2014). Decrease of a specific biomarker of collagen degradation in osteoarthritis, coll2-1, by treatment with highly bioavailable curcumin during an exploratory clinical trial. *BMC Complementary and Alternative Medicine, 14*, 159.

Jenkins, D.J.A., Spence, J.D., Giovannucci, E.L., Kim, Y., Josse, R., Vieth, R., Mejia, S.B., Viguiliouk, E., Nishi, S., Sahye-Pudaruth, S., Paquette, M., Patel, D., Mitchell, S., Kavanagh, M., Tsirakis, T., Bachiri, L., Maran, A., Umatheva, N., McKay, T., … Sievenpiper, J.L. (2018). Supplemental vitamins and minerals for CVD prevention and treatment. *Journal of the American College of Cardiology, 71*(22), 2570–84.

Kassoff, A., Kassoff, J., Buehler, J., Eglow, M., Kaufman, F., Mehu, M., & Crouse, V.D. (2001). A randomized, placebo-controlled, clinical trial of high-dose supplementation with vitamins C and E, beta carotene, and zinc for age-related macular degeneration and vision loss: AREDS report No. 8. *Archives of Ophthalmology, 119*(10), 1417–1436.

Klein, E.A., Thompson, I.M., Tangen, C.M., et al. (2011, October 12). Vitamin E and the risk of prostate cancer: The selenium and vitamin E cancer prevention trial. *Journal of the American Medical Association, 306*(14), 1549–1556. doi:10.1001/jama.2011.1437

Kornblut, A. E., and Wilson, D. (2005, April 17). How one pill escaped the list of controlled steroids. *The New York Times.* https://www.nytimes.com/2005/04/17/us/how-one-pill-escaped-the-list-of-controlled-steroids.html

Lonn, E., Bosch, J., Yusuf, S., Sheridan, P., Pogue, J., Arnold, J.M., Ross, C., Arnold, A., Sleight, P., Probstfield, J., Dagenais, G. R., & HOPE and HOPE-TOO Trial Investigators. (2005). Effects of long-term vitamin E supplementation on cardiovascular events and cancer: A randomized controlled trial. *Journal of the American Medical Association, 293*(11), 1338–47.

Meyerowitz-Katz, G. (2017, August 14). *No, turmeric is not a cancer cure.* Observer. http://observer.com/2017/08/turmeric-curcuminoids-cancer-cure/

Moulite, M. (2018, August 7). *Are the health benefits of turmeric too good to be true?* CNN. https://www.cnn.com/2018/08/07/health/turmeric-benefits-explainer/index.html

Myers, S. (2015). *Clinical trials: Two-thirds of supplement companies support research.* Natural Products Insider. https://www.naturalproductsinsider.com/claims/clinical-trials-two-thirds-supplement-companies-support-research

NIH Consortium for Advancing Research on Botanical and Other Natural Products (CARBON) Program. https://ods.od.nih.gov/Research/Dietary_Supplement_Research_Centers.aspx

Office of Dietary Supplements. (2001). *Evidence-based review program.* National Institutes of Health, Office of Dietary Supplements. https://ods.od.nih.gov/Research/Evidence-Based_Review_Program.aspx

Pittler, M.H., & Ernst, E. (2004). Dietary supplements for body-weight reduction: A systematic review. *The American Journal of Clinical Nutrition, 79*(4), 529–536.

Riemann, D., Baglioni, C., Bassetti, C., Bjorvatn, B., Dolenc Groselj, L., Ellis, J.G., Espie, C.A., Garcia-Borreguero, D., Gjerstad, M., Gonçalves, M., Hertenstein, E., Jansson-Fröjmark, M., Jennum,

P.J., Leger, D., Nissen, C., Parrino, L., Paunio, T., Pevernagie, D., Verbraecken, J., ... Spiegelhalder, K. (2017). European guideline for the diagnosis and treatment of insomnia. *J Sleep Res.*, *26*(6), 675–700. doi: 10.1111/jsr.12594. Epub 2017 Sep 5. PMID: 28875581.

Small, G.W., Siddarth, P., Li, Z., Miller, K.J., Ercoli, L., Emerson, N.D., Martinez, J., et al. (2018). Memory and brain amyloid and tau effects of a bioavailable form of curcumin in non-demented adults: A double-blind, placebo-controlled 18-month trial. *American Journal of Geriatric Psychiatry*, *26*(3), 266–77.

Sorkin, B., Kuszak, A., Bloss, G., Fukagawa, N., Jafari, M., Walters, M., et al. (2020). (Office of Dietary Supplement NIH Working Group). Improving natural product research translation: From source to clinical trial. *The FASEB Journal*, *34*, 41–65.

Swanson, C.A. (2002). Suggested guidelines for articles about botanical dietary supplements. *The American Journal of Clinical Nutrition*, *75*(1), 8–10.

Turmeric for Health. (2016). *20 benefits of turmeric in fighting cancer naturally*. Turmeric for Health. https://www.turmericforhealth.com/turmeric -benefits/turmeric-for-cancer

Vivekananthan, D.P., Penn, M.S., Sapp, S.K., Hsu, A., & Topol, E.J. (2003). Use of antioxidant vitamins for the prevention of cardiovascular disease: Meta-analysis of randomised trials. *Lancet*, *361*(9374), 2017–23.

Wang, M. T. M., Gamble, G., Bolland, M.J., & Grey, A. (2014). Press releases issued by supplements industry organisations and non-industry organisations in response to publication of clinical research findings: A case-control study. *PLOS ONE*, *9*(7), e101533.

Wolsko, P. M., Solondz, D. K., Phillips, R. S., Schachter, S. C., & Eisenberg, D. M. (2005). Lack of herbal supplement characterization in published randomized controlled trials. *American Journal of Medicine*, *118*(10), 1087–1093.

Woolston, C. (2012, May 19). Are raspberry ketones a 'miracle' fat burner? Dr. Oz weighs in. *Los Angeles Times*. Recovered from: http://

articles.latimes.com/2012/may/19/health/la-he-raspberry-ketone
-20120519

Zajak, A. (2010, September 8). FDA warns green tea makers against
health claims. *Los Angeles Times*. Retrieved from: http://articles
.latimes.com/2010/sep/08/nation/la-na-fda-tea-20100908

CHAPTER 5

THE POWER OF MEDIA TO BRAINWASH THE PUBLIC

STORY

A few years ago, I received a text message from a friend asking me about the effectiveness of *Garcinia cambogia* for weight loss. She had heard on *The Dr. Oz Show* that *Garcinia* is very effective for weight loss and that Dr. Oz himself had called it a miracle pill for weight loss. This extract comes from a fruit grown in Asia, India, and Africa, and those who sell it purport it to be an excellent appetite suppressant. Bottles were flying off the shelves—my friend wasn't the only one who was intrigued.

I did a literature search on the effectiveness of *Garcinia* for weight loss, and although I found the fruit to be safe, except for reports of occasional nausea and headaches, I could not find any scientific evidence in clinical studies that proved it to be effective for weight loss. While I was performing my search, I also found a class action lawsuit against Dr. Oz, which stated that, despite his glowing endorsement, "all credible scientific evidence" proves that *Garcinia cambogia* does not work. In 2014, Dr. Oz appeared before a congressional hearing for promoting *Garcinia* as a miracle pill for weight loss, and he admitted that the fruit's track record does not have enough "scientific muster to present as facts." A representative for *The Dr. Oz Show* has since said the lawsuit is an attack on free speech (Konstantanides, 2016).

I am a big fan of freedom of speech. But I also believe that celebrities like Dr. Oz who host popular TV shows on major broadcast networks have the responsibility to do their homework, research their topic, and make evidence-based recommendations. I also believe that celebrities should be transparent about receiving payments or any other type of incentives for endorsing products.

THE DOCTOR IS ALWAYS IN: MEDIA AS A PRIMARY SOURCE OF HEALTH INFORMATION

What is the first thing you do when you have a question about your health, or that of a family member? If you pull out your cell phone or head to your computer, you are part of a quiet revolution that is taking place. People are gathering information to help them make decisions about their health differently than in the past. Of those who regularly use the internet, 80% report looking up medical information for themselves or others. A recent national survey showed that this is one of the primary uses of the internet, right after checking email and researching a product or a service (Weaver, 2013).

In the past, physicians were often the gatekeepers of most medical knowledge and choices; today, it is common for patients to come to their doctors with requests based on information they have found by themselves online or from magazine articles and television shows. In 2015, WebMD, a for-profit health website, reported that their website had 74 million visitors each month (WebMD Health Services, 2015)! The fallout of this information revolution is, of course, complicated. Wonderfully, more medical information is available to more people than ever before; but troublingly, the quality of this information is extremely variable, and the average person may not always be well-equipped to judge it well.

MEDIA AND THE MARKETING OF DIETARY SUPPLEMENTS: "SCIENCE" AND CELEBRITY

This change in the way we use technology has opened our lives to a multitude of voices trying to influence our health, and these voices are one of the key factors that shape people's understanding of dietary supplements and drive the sales of the supplement industry.

For instance, in one study, interviews were conducted to learn what factors contributed to people's choice to take supplements. Although respondents gave a variety of specific reasons, from hoping to prevent cancer to boosting their immune system to concerns about a poor diet, there was one common thread among supplement users: The interviews revealed that, indeed, there is a significant shift in the information-gathering process that individuals go through as they make decisions about their health. Though people trusted their doctor the most and were very likely to take any supplements advised by their physician, the media was consistently mentioned as a source of influence. And the more supplements a person took, the more confidence they placed in media as a trustworthy information source. Those taking the most supplements also reported that they felt it was important to "self-educate" about supplement usage. Younger participants also expressed more confidence than older ones in their ability to independently gain good health recommendations from media (Peters et al., 2003).

The Pew Research Center reports that about 35% of Americans head to the internet—"Dr. Google"—to self-diagnose their symptoms (Fox, 2013). This is a widespread problem from the viewpoint of physicians. Increased patient knowledge is an excellent thing, but self-diagnosis and treatment based on bad information can be life-threatening (Peters et al., 2003).

From a marketing perspective, it makes sense to lean into this phenomenon. Companies are trying to capture the "self-directed" health consumer by presenting the pitches for their products in ways that closely mimic research. As the above study found, it is not unusual to see what are essentially paid ads that masquerade as academic and scientific reports or health forums.

In August of 2017, the FTC and the State of Maine successfully brought charges against a supplement maker that used deceptive advertising to sell its wares. The company used thirty-minute radio ads designed to sound like educational talks to sell a supplement that claimed to be clinically proven to reverse memory loss. In the end, the "scientific expert" billed by the company as endorsing its product was shown to have never investigated the product's efficacy—but he was getting a cut of its sales (Federal Trade Commission, 2017b).

A Florida-based supplement seller was found to not only be making deceptive claims about a series of supplements that they produced (one for weight loss, another for curing colds, and yet another for treating HIV symptoms), but also of making a fake certification site that supposedly gave their products an independent "Certified Ethical Site" verification (Federal Trade Commission, 2017a). Too often, unscrupulous supplement companies are greedy wolves wearing pseudoscientific sheep's clothing.

This "scientific styling" of supplement marketing makes sense because, just as pharmaceutical companies are known for spending a fortune trying to woo doctors and consumers, the supplement industry must make its sales by directly appealing to consumers, many of whom are looking for scientific cues to make their purchases.

McKinsey & Company, an international management consulting firm, put together an insightful report forecasting the future of the dietary supplement industry, written specifically for investors and entrepreneurs. They found that aging populations play a role in supporting sales, as does the increased public interest in preventive healthcare and wellness. Center stage, though, is the rise of the self-directed consumer. The report writes that "many supplement purchases are the result of consumers taking their health into their own hands, not the direct advice of a doctor." The report notes that some 70% of

Americans use the internet in connection with their health, commonly gaining information before and after their doctors' appointments (Teichner & Lesko, 2013).

Many dietary supplement manufacturers have responded to this new normal by giving consumers what they want: easily attainable health "information" and the perceived tools of self-diagnosis that point back to their products.

By no means is it impossible for companies to present valid data backing their products' efficacy, nor do I wish to imply that they all hope to hoodwink their customers. Thankfully, that is not the case. The problem I hope to highlight is that it can be very difficult to distinguish between information that is coming from a paid marketing firm versus an independent research team. This is a challenge that is unlikely to go away anytime soon, and while the FDA and the FTC chase false claims, the best protection is simply consumer awareness. As we noted in past chapters, sources matter!

The marketing report doesn't end there, and neither does the story of how media drives supplement sales. At times consumers are influenced by what they perceive to be reliable health information, but sales trends also show that many purchases and health choices are instinctual. Fads are a critical (but unruly) driver of sales, and those fads are often sparked by the example of celebrities. Sometimes this influence is wholly spontaneous and could be beneficial, as in 2005 when it was revealed that the popular Australian pop singer Kylie Minogue was diagnosed with breast cancer, causing mammograms to rise by 40% in four Australian states. In 2000, Katie Couric had the NBC's *Today Show* cameras follow her through her colonoscopy appointment. Sure enough, within a month, four hundred American endoscopists recorded an increase in colorectal cancer screenings of 21% (Hoffman & Tan, 2013). In 2012, Angelina Jolie wrote a public letter in *The New York Times* about her decision to have a preventive double mastectomy after genetic testing showed that she had a high chance of one day developing breast cancer, and, despite the statistical rarity of Jolie's situation, women flocked to take the same genetic test. A national study of women with health insurance found a 64% increase in testing in the fifteen days after the editorial was published. This study noted that while some good may come from raising awareness about a particular condition, unnecessary panic, the rapid spread of misinformation, and confusion also seem to be a corollary to celebrity health events like these (Desai & Anupam, 2016).

The endorsements of famous figures can have a marked effect on the public, but the major media powerhouses are wellness celebrities. The McKinsey report found that "Health-conscious media celebrities such as Dr. Oz, Deepak Chopra, and Jillian Michaels have always had a major impact on [supplement] sales because consumers trust their advice" (Teichner & Lesko, 2013). So, if Dr. Oz mentions the power of *Garcinia cambogia* as a miracle pill for weight loss or his favorite brand of fiber supplements on air, stores can see their shelves stripped bare of the product in twenty-four hours (Walton, 2011). The commitment on the part of consumers doesn't always stick, but at least in the short term the influence of these recommendations is palpable.

We will return to Dr. Oz and the unprecedented reach of wellness celebrities, but before we explore this phenomenon, it's worth asking: Why do famous people exert so much influence? And are we somehow more susceptible to this influence today than in the past?

The Halo and the Herd: The Psychology of Celebrity Influence

The oldest marketing trick in the book is positive association: Take something that people already love and set alongside it what you want to sell, hoping that the good feelings toward the former will rub off on the latter (Till et al., 2008). In the world of psychology, this is called classical conditioning, and it works. Since the 1950s, Wheaties cereal boxes have shared their name with a host of Olympians and star athletes, each of whom successfully reinforced the image that Wheaties was indeed the "Breakfast of Champions." Time and again, celebrity endorsements of products has paid off—especially if the product and the celebrity have some kind of congruence or shared trait (Choi & Rifon, 2012). Understandably then, health and fitness celebrities such as Jillian Michaels, famous as a trainer from the TV show *The Biggest Loser*, have an enormous impact on what health products and practices are in vogue.

Not only do celebrity choices and endorsements help to create a positive view of a product by association (sometimes called the halo effect), but this practice also triggers what is popularly known in texting lingo as FOMO: fear of missing out. When presented with another person's experience or choice, our minds must evaluate whether or not we too would benefit from the same thing. Commercials and ads all exist for this single purpose: to convince us that we *are* missing out, that our lives would be better and healthier and happier if we just had whatever it is that is on offer.

Sociologists devote great attention to "herd behavior," the common reflex that leads us to follow others, and the variety of elusive ways the group shapes the individual. A classic example is adopting similar body language to those around you. If everyone in a group has their arms crossed, you might find yourself in the same position without even thinking about it. There is a certain level of pain or discomfort experienced when we don't follow the rest of the group, especially if we perceive that group as successful or desirable (Till et al., 2008). In the case of celebrity endorsements, we see these natural human feelings and responses leveraged to the max. Someone who is immensely successful is making a choice, and we are presented with a chance to partake in a little piece of that success ourselves, or alternately, be doomed to fall behind.

Of course, all of this logic is usually unconscious and can take place in the blink of an eye. We are not wholly controlled by these impulses, but sales numbers show that we are not immune to them either.

Anecdotes and Star Power: The Influence of Social Media on Purchases

Such marketing strategies, which are designed to manipulate age-old human impulses and turn them into purchases, have been going on for as long as people have been buying and selling things. What is new, and of great significance for the rise of the dietary supplement industry, are the changes that we see with the advent of the internet, television advertisements, and modern social media.

Why is this so important? And how has it amplified the influence of celebrities of all kinds on public discussion and understanding of health? The bottom line is that we are coming into contact with more media than ever before, and the nature of that media makes it easy for celebrities of all stripes to influence our perceptions of what it takes to be well.

In the past, access to conventional media was restricted. Celebrities were often the stars, but the stages that they appeared on were relatively few (films controlled by studios, TV shows controlled by major broadcasting networks, newspapers, billboards, etc.). But with the birth of social media networks in the late 1990s, celebrities gained unlimited stages on which to connect with the public—in fact, some are famous solely *because* of social media. Platforms like Twitter, Facebook, and Instagram are free, and rather than marketers strategizing to find ways for consumers to encounter their campaigns, people seek out their favorite celebrities' social media outlets of their own accord.

As of 2021, Deepak Chopra, champion of his own brand of alternative medicine, has 2.3 million followers on his Instagram account and 3 million followers on his Twitter account; Gwyneth Paltrow, actress-turned-health-entrepreneur, has 7.5 million followers on her Instagram account; and Dr. Oz has five million people and counting following his Facebook page. All of these social media sites act as new stages, freely available twenty-four hours a day, which public figures can utilize to increase their contact with fans and followers.

The informality of social media can also increase people's feeling of closeness to famous individuals.

In 2018, seven out of ten Americans—70%—used social media (up dramatically from the just 5% of American adults who used it in 2005). And not only do the majority of Americans seek out these platforms, but they do so with predictable frequency. The Pew Research Center found that "for many users, social media is part of their daily routine. Roughly three-quarters of Facebook users—and around six-in-ten Instagram users—visit these sites at least once a day" (Pew Research Center, 2019).

This all adds up to a world in which there is ample opportunity for celebrities to shape people's understanding of health and influence their practices and purchases. Most of the time, celebrities aren't forthcoming about the kinds of paychecks they receive to endorse products. But in the case of social media, sometimes we can follow the algorithms to find the money. *The Economist* reports that a company called Captiv8, which identifies potential social media influencers for companies hoping to advertise, says that "someone with 3m-7m followers can charge, on average, $187,500 for a post on YouTube, $93,750 for a post on Facebook and $75,000 for a post on Instagram or Snapchat." By law, even though these ads appear on personal accounts, they must be identified as ads (you'll often see "#ad" at the end of the post). For a site such as Instagram, which began in 2011, its use as a very lucrative endorsement platform has skyrocketed in its short existence. In 2017, some 400,000 sponsored ads were being posted each month (*The Economist*, 2016).

Instagram hosts an especially high concentration of supplement ads, many of which are beauty-oriented. Because middle- and upper-class women are the primary buyers of supplements and Instagram is most popular among that demographic, this is a match made in marketing heaven (Wischhover, 2018).

Timothy Caulfield's book *Is Gwyneth Paltrow Wrong About Everything? How the Famous Sell Us Elixirs of Health, Beauty & Happiness* argues that something like an Instagram photo can be a very powerful motivator, and that every snapshot of a celebrity with a particular product is an anecdote in itself. It's a tiny, casual story with a tantalizing subconscious promise: "You can be me, too!" Stories will always be relatable and tangible in a way that numbers and generalities cannot match (Caulfield, 2016). Social media posts, which are almost always informal cell phone "selfies" of the celebrity with the product, perfectly reinforce this façade of genuine closeness, and by extension, trustworthiness.

Celebrity Wellness Experts

Endorsements and product placement ads are money-making machines, but the most influential media voices of all are health celebrities—those who make wellness their full-time job. Here I will share two of many examples.

Dr. Oz

The premier "celebri-doc" is no doubt Mehmet Oz, who was first introduced on Oprah in 2004, then went on to star in his own show in 2009. In its prime, *The Dr. Oz Show* had 3.4 million viewers tuning in every day. Nicknamed "America's Doctor," this heart-surgeon-turned-TV-personality continues to enjoy immense popularity. He has proven to be a talented showman, using fire on stage as an analogy for burning away belly fat; inviting former First Lady Michelle Obama to come and dance with him to sponsor her "Let's Move!" national fitness campaign; and in each episode offering engaging advice on physiology, nutrition, and common health problems. It has made for very good TV for nine seasons and counting.

The show has become famous for catapulting health products onto the bestsellers list (known in the retail business as "The Dr. Oz Effect"). For instance, after featuring neti pots on his show, internet searches of the product increased by 42,000%, and neti pot sales by 12,000% (Bootsman et al., 2014). The neti pot is a nasal irrigation system that uses a saline or saltwater solution. According to the FDA, improper use of a neti pot can cause infection due to use of tap water to clean it. Some tap waters contain bacteria that are normally killed by the acidity of our stomach, but in our nasal cavities, they can grow and cause serious infections (FDA, 2017). Similarly, after Oz presented green coffee bean extract and raspberry ketones as supplements that had miraculous fat-burning effects, Google search history shows that the terms, which had virtually no searches prior, shot up overnight. Each time the episodes re-aired, a resurgence in searches (and we can assume in sales) occurred (Bootsman et al., 2014). Very few people are able to direct the public's attention on matters of health and wellness to this degree, or influence health product and supplement sales so radically. The fans of Dr. Oz are many, but so are his critics, who have accused him of presenting "miracle" products to his audience that in truth have little or insufficient scientific research behind them.

In 2014, a team of qualified health researchers did an observational study of two of the most popular health talk shows on air, *The Dr. Oz Show* and *The Doctors*. Reviewing eighty episodes, they listed every health claim made in each one, from the mundane to the bizarre, and set out to review the scientific research behind these claims. In all, 180 recommendations were put to the test. The results? Fifty-four percent of those recommendations were backed by scientific research. In the case of *The Dr. Oz Show*, "Evidence supported 46%, contradicted 15%, and was not found for 39%" of his health claims. Given those numbers, even assuming a wide margin of error, the article's conclusion seems almost unnecessary: "Consumers should be skeptical about any recommendations provided on television medical talk shows, as details are limited and only a third to one half of recommendations are based on believable or somewhat believable evidence" (Korownyk et al., 2014).

The U.S. Congress has much the same view. As I mentioned at the beginning of this chapter, in 2014, a congressional hearing was called by the Subcommittee on Consumer Protection, Product Safety, and Insurance, and Dr. Oz was invited along with several other physicians to discuss the problem. The broad purpose of the hearing was to gather information and testimony regarding how to best protect consumers from potentially dangerous weight-loss products, but it quickly turned into a very pointed critique of the way that Dr. Oz used his considerable influence. Senator Claire McCaskill (D-MO), while noting that Oz regularly gave good basic advice on the importance of a healthy lifestyle, was disturbed that Oz, a trained physician, could embrace so many "miracle" cures. She told Oz, "I'm concerned that you are melding medical advice, news, and entertainment in a way that harms consumers" (U.S. Senate, 2014).

One infamous example is the green coffee bean extract craze he triggered in 2012. With characteristic charisma, he opened his show with the announcement that "this little bean has scientists saying that they have found a magic weight-loss cure for every body type." While showcasing a montage of shrinking bellies, the audience was told that a groundbreaking new study revealed that you could lose 17 pounds in 22 weeks by taking the supplement, without changing any of your eating habits or exercising. Oz brought on a guest star, Lindsey Duncan, to explain the properties of this "Dieter's Secret Weapon." Duncan, presenting himself as a naturopathic doctor, was in reality connected to a marketing firm that was itching to make a fortune on the extract. Major news outlets followed the fallout of the episode: Stores couldn't re-stock green coffee bean extract fast enough. Millions of dollars in sales were made across the country (Philip, 2015).

The craze received so much attention that the FTC decided to investigate and quickly found the data used in the clinical trial to be unreliable—in their words, "seriously flawed." A legal complaint was issued against Applied Food Science, Inc., which sponsored and published the study (U.S. District Court, 2014). The FTC showed that the trial, which took place in India, was filled with irregularities: conflicting data sets, conspicuously tampered-with entries concerning participants' weight, and other damaging omissions. Researchers had been paid to polish the original study, which was not of publishable quality. The FTC investigation led to the authors' retraction of the paper, and in 2015, Duncan's company had to pay $9 million to those who bought the product based on their deceptive advertising (Federal Trade Commission, 2015).

Dr. Oz was not involved in this coverup, but he was gullible enough to host its perpetrators on his show. He has since removed the episode from his website and issued a statement that gently seems to chalk up the mistake to the scientific process of trial and error, rather than a deleterious error in his own judgment (Dr. Oz Show, 2014).

Most of the lawsuits and scams associated with his name are in this same vein: parasite industries poised to jump the moment that Oz mentions something on his show, waging aggressive internet campaigns that purport to be selling Dr. Oz's products. To his credit, Dr. Oz regularly warns his viewers against such scams. However, he also uses his megaphone to start these trends in the first place.

Gwyneth Paltrow's "Goop"

In 2016, actress Gwyneth Paltrow expanded her lifestyle brand into supplement sales and wellness products, beginning Goop Wellness. The first day, she sold $100,000 in products. One year later, the watchdog group Truth in Advertising (TINA.org) submitted a letter to her company. On her website they found fifty unsubstantiated health claims (Truth in Advertising, 2017). After Goop made minimal changes, Truth in Advertising filed a complaint requesting a formal investigation of the company by California regulators. Paltrow, whose products included something called "Crystal Harmonics," which was supposed to treat infertility, brushed off the criticism in an interview as an assault on women's autonomy (Szklarski, 2017).

Dr. Jen Gunter, an obstetrician and gynecologist, criticized several of Paltrow's recommendations and products in her personal blog, concerned especially about the products aimed at women's fertility and sexual enhancement. She told *The New York Times*, "I'd just write it off as crazy except some people are going to follow this advice and waste a lot of money" (Rosman, 2017). The luxe website and bohemian product names belie the hard facts of the matter: If these supplements are bought and consumed in hopes of treating something as devastating as infertility, the science had better be there to justify the credit card bill.

Interestingly, the packaging of Goop's dietary supplements is not ingredient-focused (a trend that the McKinsey report says is picking up speed), but instead cutely taps into the idea that you can buy a certain lifestyle or feeling. The product "High School Genes," individual packets of vitamins that are to be taken daily, costs $90 for one month's worth, and though a snapshot of the supplements' ingredients is included on the webpage (nothing out of the ordinary), the entire description of the product fails to mention a single ingredient. Like other luxury items, it is trying to sell you an experience—a return to your younger days. But supplements are not designer jeans: No matter how chic the presentation, dietary supplements have a real pharmacological effect on our bodies.

CONCLUSION

Whenever presented with slick websites and scientific-sounding descriptions, or with the stories and endorsements of the rich and famous, practice common sense. There is a lot of money to be made selling supplements, and marketers are doing their best to make it whatever way they can. There may be scientifically validated dietary supplements that will benefit your health, but that will depend entirely on your story and your health status, not someone else's. We need to learn to discriminate between misleading claims and statistics on one hand and valid scientific evidence on the other hand. What does *your* body truly need? Chapter 7 is my guide to the tested-and-true methods for identifying deficiencies.

TAKEAWAYS

When you look for information about health and dietary supplements on the internet, make sure to find the following information:

- Who is operating, presenting, or sponsoring the website? Is the website run by reputable organizations such as the Food and Drug Administration (FDA), the National Institute of Health (NIH), the Office of Dietary Supplements (ODS), a reputable university, or a trustworthy nonprofit organization? These sites usually have a ".gov" or ".edu" URL extension. If this is not the case, you need to learn more about the validity of the information presented in that website. Be careful with ".org" domain names. Note that domain names are not as regularly policed as they were in the early 1990s when the internet was changing from a government entity to a commercial entity. The ".org" may not necessarily represent a nonprofit organization.

- Is the website selling any products? Most educational sites do not sell or advertise specific products. You have to be careful because some sites may appear as educational and then list links to scientific papers that simply represent pseudoscience.

- When a site lists a scientific publication, find out if that paper was published in a peer-reviewed scientific journal and determine who sponsored the research. Who are the authors? What are their affiliations? Do they work for the company that sponsored the research, or are they scientists working in universities and government organizations like NIH and FDA?

- When reading testimonials about dietary supplements by celebrities, find out if the testimonial is an ad (look for #ad). Testimonials are simply anecdotes, and they are not science. As we learned, it is human nature to be interested in other people's stories, but we need to do our due diligence.

- Consult with your physician and other healthcare providers before starting to take a dietary supplement.

ADDITIONAL RESOURCES

- Information regarding dietary supplement recalls: U.S. Food & Drug Administration.

  https://www.fda.gov

- A basic overview of dietary supplements facts: National Institute of Health Office of Dietary Supplements.

  https://ods.od.nih.gov

- Information about deceptive and false advertisements: Truth in Advertising.

  www.truthinadvertising.org

REFERENCES

Bootsman, N., Blackburn, D.F., & Taylor, J. (2014). The Oz craze: The effect of pop culture media on health care. *Canadian Pharmacists Journal, 147*(2), 80–82.

Caulfield, T. (2016). *Is Gwyneth Paltrow wrong about everything?: How the famous sell us elixirs of health, beauty & happiness.* Beacon Press.

Choi, S.M., & Rifon, N.J. (2012). It is a match: The impact of congruence between celebrity image and consumer ideal self on endorsement effectiveness. *Psychology and Marketing, 29*(9), 639–650.

Desai, S., & Anupam, J.B. (2016). Do celebrity endorsements matter? Observational study of BRCA gene testing and mastectomy rates after Angelina Jolie's *New York Times* editorial. *BMJ, 355*, i6357. https://www.bmj.com/content/355/bmj.i6357.

Dr. Oz Show. (2014). *Recent developments regarding green coffee extract.* Retrieved from: https://www.doctoroz.com/page/recent-developments-regarding-green-coffee-extract

Federal Trade Commission. (2015, January 26). *Press release: Marketer who promoted a green coffee bean weight-loss supplement agrees to settle FTC charges.* Federal Trade Commission. https://www.ftc.gov/news-events/press-releases/2015/01/marketer-who-promoted-green-coffee-bean-weight-loss-supplement

———. (2017b, August 23). *Three dietary supplement marketers settle FTC, Maine AG charges.* Federal Trade Commission. https://www.ftc.gov/news-events/press-releases/2017/08/three-dietary-supplement-marketers-settle-ftc-maine-ag-charges

———. (2017a, November 20). Florida-based supplement sellers settle FTC false advertising charges. Federal Trade Commission. https://www.ftc.gov/news-events/press-releases/2017/11/florida-based-supplement-sellers-settle-ftc-false-advertising

Fox, Susannah. (2013, December 17). *What ails America? Dr. Google can tell you.* Pew Research Center: Fact Tank. http://www.pewresearch.org/fact-tank/2013/12/17/what-ails-america-dr-google-can-tell-you

Hoffman, S.J., & Tan, C. (2013). Following celebrities' medical advice: Meta-narrative analysis. *BMJ, 347*, f7151.

Konstantanides, A. (2016, February 3). *Dr. Oz sued for weight loss supplement he claimed was a 'revolutionary fat buster with no exercises, no diet, no effort.'* Daily Mail. https://www.dailymail.co.uk/news/article-3430075/Dr -Oz-sued-weight-loss-supplement-Garcinia-Cambogia.html

Korownyk, C., Kolber, M.R., McCormack, J.P., Lam, V., Overbo, K., Cotton, C., Finley, C.R., Turgeon, R.D., Garrison, S., Lindblad, A.J., Banh, H.L., Campbell-Scherer, D., Vandermeer, B., & Allan, G.M. (2014). Televised medical talk shows—What they recommend and the evidence to support their recommendations: A prospective observational study. *BMJ, 349*, g7346.

Peters, C.O., Shelton, J., & Sharma, P. (2003). An investigation of factors that influence the consumption of dietary supplements. *Health Marketing Quarterly, 21*(1–2), 113–35.

Pew Research Center. (2019, June 12). *Social media fact sheet.* Pew Research Center. http://www.pewinternet.org/fact-sheet/social-media/

Philip, A. (2015, January 28). How a fake doctor made millions from 'the Dr. Oz Effect' and a bogus weight-loss supplement. *The Washington Post.* https://www.washingtonpost.com/news/morning-mix/wp /2015/01/28/how-a-fake-doctor-made-millions-from-the-dr-oz -effect-and-a-bogus-weight-loss-supplement/?noredirect=on&utm _term=.ff7109e19463

Rosman, K. (2017, July 29). A doctor gives Gwyneth Paltrow's Goop an examination. *The New York Times.* https://www.nytimes.com/2017 /07/29/style/goop-gwyneth-paltrow-dr-jen-gunter.html

Szklarski, C. (2017, September 4). *Timothy Caulfield is pleased about renewed attack on Gwyneth Paltrow's Goop.* Huffington Post. https://www .huffingtonpost.ca/2018/01/09/gwyneth-paltrow-coffee-enema _a_23328873/

Teichner, W., & Lesko, M. (2013, December). *Cashing in on the booming market for dietary supplements.* McKinsey & Company. https://www

.mckinsey.com/business-functions/marketing-and-sales/our-insights/cashing-in-on-the-booming-market-for-dietary-supplements

The Economist. (2016, October 17). *Celebrities' endorsement earnings on social media*. The Economist. https://www.economist.com/graphic-detail/2016/10/17/celebrities-endorsement-earnings-on-social-media

Till, B.D., Stanley, S.M., & Priluck, R. (2008). Classical conditioning and celebrity endorsers: An examination of belongingness and resistance to extinction. *Psychology and Marketing, 25*(2), 179–196.

Truth in Advertising. (2017, August 22). Tina.org *takes Gwyneth Paltrow's Goop-Y health claims to regulators*. Truth in Advertising. https://www.truthinadvertising.org/tina-takes-goop-claims-to-regulators/

United States District Court for the Western District of Texas. (2014). *Federal Trade Commission v. Applied Food Sciences, Inc.* Federal Trade Commission. https://www.ftc.gov/system/files/documents/cases/140908afscmpt.pdf

United States Food and Drug Administration. (2017, January 23). *Is rinsing your sinuses with neti pots safe?* Department of Health and Human Services, Federal Drug Administration. https://www.fda.gov/consumers/consumer-updates/rinsing-your-sinuses-neti-pots-safe

United States Senate. (2014, June 17). *Hearing of the committee on commerce, science and transportation: Protecting consumers from false and deceptive advertising of weight-loss products, June 17, 2014*. Retrieved from: https://www.gpo.gov/fdsys/pkg/CHRG-113shrg92998/html/CHRG-113shrg92998.htm

Walton, A.G. (2011, June 6). *The Oz effect: medicine or marketing?* Forbes. https://www.forbes.com/sites/alicegwalton/2011/06/06/the-oz-effect-medicine-or-marketing/#153175eb3233

Weaver, J. (2013). *More people search for health online*. NBC News. http://www.nbcnews.com/id/3077086/t/more-people-search-health-online/#.XFYT0FxKhPZ

WebMD Health Services. (2015). Retrieved from: https://www.webmdhealthservices.com/product/webmd-content/

Wischhover, C. (2018, April 9). *Vitamins for your hair, nails, and skin are everywhere on Instagram. Don't fall for them.* Vox. https://www.vox.com/2018/4/9/17199164/beauty-vitamin-collagen-turmeric-biotin

CHAPTER 6

THE TRUTH ABOUT PET SUPPLEMENTS

STORY

I became aware of this dimension of the supplement market thanks to a phone call from an old friend. She was in Costco, tunneling her way through the towering aisle of pet products, when she saw a dietary supplement that claimed that it could treat arthritis in dogs. "Does it work?" she asked me. Her dog was over ten years old, and he was moving slowly. Of course, she wanted to take the best possible care of him. However, the supplement, even in bulk, was expensive. Would it work? Was it entirely safe? I told her: "I don't know if it will help, but I can try to find out."

I understood her situation and was sympathetic: I once had a beautiful Italian greyhound named Bisou. My son grew up with her, we all adored her, and we bent over backwards to get her anything she needed. She truly was part of the family.

THE EVER-EXPANDING MARKET FOR PET PRODUCTS

Thus far, we have learned that most American adults take a dietary supplement daily, and that supplement consumption is on the rise for many age groups, including the elderly, young adults, and children. But the trend does not stop there. Increasingly, people are buying supplements and giving them to their pets as well.

To be honest, when I spoke with my friend, I didn't know what an interesting world I was promising to investigate. First, I found that, despite the economic recession of the late 2000s, pet ownership is higher now than in the 1990s: In 2017, 68% of American households owned a pet—up from 56% in 1998 (American Pet Products Association, 2017). Taking care of all those pets comes with a sizable price tag: $69 billion was spent on the purchase and maintenance of pets in 2017, with the number one spending category being food (American Pet Products Association, 2017). Pet dietary supplements are also becoming a common expenditure. Currently, "a third of all U.S. households with dogs use supplements, as do about a fifth of households with cats" (Burns, 2017).

Not only do more households have pets, but those that do tend to see their pets differently than they would have fifty years ago. Pets are now an integral part of the family, and market researchers emphasize the dawn of the "fur baby" and "pet parents" (Olivo, 2017). From a business perspective, this inspires endless opportunities to make a profit helping people care for and enjoy the pets that they are so very attached to. Just as people worry about their own health, they are also concerned about their pets' health, which has led to a lucrative market for specialty "health" foods and supplemented treats.

If you live in an urban area, you have probably witnessed some manifestation of these pet-specialty boutiques and products firsthand. Especially in the more affluent parts of the country, pet owners like to extend versions of their own favorite luxuries to their animals. Here in Orange County, there are pet bakeries, such as "Top Dog Barkery," in Newport Beach, famous for making personalized birthday cakes for pooches and throwing "Pup Showers" when someone's furry friend is expecting. Bacon and peanut butter usually feature heavily in their offerings. (Not aware that the "Top Dog Barkery" was dedicated to pet treats, the first time I passed by it, I walked in and bought a small, tasty-looking chocolate cookie—and ate it myself. It smelled and tasted like dried chicken. Who knows what the employees must have thought!)

All across the country, the pet luxury business is booming as never before. In New York City, you can book a $200-a-night pet hotel suite that features full-sized beds and "dog-friendly programming" (Rogers, 2017). What that might be, I can only imagine. People might see this as an expression of a deep love for animals that is heartwarming, or the more skeptical may find such expenditures frivolous. Either way, if your cat has a Tiffany & Co. collar or you buy Fido some "Doggles" (specially designed dog sunglasses), there is no harm done to the animal. But that is not true when it comes to purchases that affect the diet of pets. Here, just as with human supplements, even though the word "healthy" might be plastered all over the product, there may be no hard, scientific evidence that it is going to create a better quality of life for your pet.

PET NUTRITION AND MARKETING HAZARDS

One glance at the pet food aisle reveals that health-based marketing is everywhere: exotic "superfood" ingredients (ostrich or açaí, anyone?) and "clean" non-GMO diets for pets are becoming more and more mainstream. Pet foods and supplemented products seem to be engaged in a fierce competition to prove that they are "healthier" than all the rest. This is good marketing because people are willing to spend a lot to buy what they think will give their animals optimum nutrition. A research team in London found that "nearly eight out of 10 pet owners said the quality of their pets' food is as important as their own" (Olivo, 2017). Another study from the *Journal of Psychology and Marketing* found that many dog owners are actually *more* serious about the healthiness of their pets' food than they are about what they put on their own plates: while 64.1% of dog owners rated their level of attention to their own diet as "serious" to "very serious," 78.4% said this about their pets' food (Tesfom & Birch, 2010).

Companies are responding by creating luxury pet food aimed at these concerned owners. A friend of mine, while at a dinner party, recently caught her toddler chowing down on doggy treats and instinctively panicked: "Icky! Icky!" she cried, while rushing to snatch the bag away from him. But then she examined the ingredient label: organic blueberries, organic seaweed, organic whole-wheat flour, and a smidge of organic cane sugar. She realized that the dog treats were healthier (and more expensive) than her kid's fruit snacks.

On the one hand, consumer preferences have encouraged the pet food market to invest in an admirable increase in the quality and transparency of some pet food. This is great news for everyone. But another consequence of consumer enthusiasm for healthier pets is vulnerability to predatory health-based marketing tactics. Products without any sound scientific research behind them may hide behind unwarranted claims to improve health and wellness. In some cases, companies even perpetuate health myths in order to sell their unproven products.

What kinds of potentially dangerous "health" fads do we find in pet nutrition? Some of them mimic human health trends: "Raw" diets, for instance, echo the logic of "paleo" diets for human beings. The general marketing story that we are told is that by eating a "natural" diet closer to that of our distant ancestors, we can reach a more perfect balance of health and harmony. For dogs and cats, this means returning to raw, meat-based diets.

But do such diets necessarily lead to better health? A recent study in the Netherlands that focused on 35 commercially sold raw dog food brands found a very high risk of these products containing harmful bacteria: 80% of the products contained *E. coli*; 50% were found to have species of *Listeria*; and 20% were contaminated with *Salmonella*. Two of the products had *Toxoplasma gondii*, a parasite that can infect cats and spread to people, with particular risk to pregnant women and babies. The authors suggest that the problem is severe enough to warrant special warning labels for raw pet diets (van Bree et al., 2018).

Another pet diet trend that mimics human health trends is vegetarianism for dogs. Some vegetarian dog owners have wanted their animals to also adopt a vegetarian diet. For cats to survive, they must eat meat because it contains essential nutrients for them, but, in theory, dogs can receive all their nutrition from plants. But are vegetarian diets best for dogs?

Of course, this in part depends on the exact content of a specific vegetarian diet, but the general answer is that these diets meet the nutritional needs of canines less often than conventional dog diets do. A study published in the *Journal of the American Veterinary Medical Association* evaluated vegetarian diets formulated for dogs to determine protein and amino acid concentrations and assess labeling adequacy. The researchers reported that of the twenty-four foods tested, most were not compliant with the minimum labeling standards of the Association of American Feed Control Officials Dog and Cat Food Nutrient Profiles and were nutritionally inadequate (Kanakubo et al., 2015).

Similarly, in an interview with *The New York Times*, Dr. Lisa Freeman, professor at Cummings School of Veterinary Medicine at Tufts University and a board-certified veterinary nutritionist, stated, "There were no long-term studies on the effects of vegetarian diets in dogs and just because veganism has health benefits in humans, it does not mean it is a healthier diet for dogs" (McDermott, 2017).

There is a strong incentive for pet companies to design and market their products toward human health trends. It's easy to piggyback their products on the already successful marketing campaigns in the world of human food and supplement sales.

So, for example, while gluten-free items for humans have stormed their way onto menus and store shelves, they are also becoming a key offering in pet food. There is "a strong rise in gluten-free and grain-free formulations for both dog and cat foods," according to Lu Ann Williams, a researcher with Innova Market Insights. "Overall, over one-fifth of [pet product] launches carried a gluten-free positioning, rising to nearly a quarter for dog food" (Burns, 2017). This change is taking place *not* because science has found that a quarter of all dogs suffer from gluten allergies, but simply because human health trends, driven in part by people's choices and in part by the encouragement of marketing campaigns, have spilled over onto pet products. While some people with severe allergy to gluten (celiac disease) should attempt to avoid any exposure to substances containing gluten, as long as they are not inadvertently ingesting gluten-containing products, they are not at risk.

In summer of 2018, the FDA's Center for Veterinary Medicine opened an investigation into multiple reports of canine dilated cardiomyopathy (DCM)—an enlargement of the heart that can lead to heart failure. Oddly, they found this problem occurring in breeds not usually genetically predisposed to it. The initial findings suggest that the common thread in these cases of DCM may be grain-free diets: "In each of the cases the dogs were being fed certain pet foods that listed potatoes, or multiple legumes such as peas, lentils, other 'pulses' (seeds of legumes), and their protein, starch and fiber derivatives as main ingredients." In other words, most were being fed diets labeled as "grain-free." The report concludes, "It is not yet known how these ingredients are linked to cases of DCM," but it still warns consumers to exercise caution (National Animal Supplement Council, 2018).

The New York Times followed the investigation, interviewed the stunned owners of the afflicted animals, and noted, "The possibility that expensive food, lovingly chosen, could make one's adored pet devastatingly ill is sending shudders through dog owners." One woman who had been feeding her golden retriever a grain-free diet for years before he developed DCM said that she had looked at the ingredients and thought: "It looked like something I would eat, so I thought it would be all right" (Hoffman, 2018).

Though the exact link between DCM and diet has not yet been uncovered, the collective angst of these dog owners can still serve to remind us of an important lesson: It is always possible that a product perceived as "healthier" is actually harmful when it does not match the real nutritional needs of a specific person (or, in this case, canine). Advertising often implies what it cannot prove, and it then generalizes when a specific assessment is called for. Dr. Freeman states that, because of the many "myths and misperceptions" surrounding pet food, it is all too easy for consumers to unknowingly "take a step in the wrong direction when the marketing outpaces the science" (Freeman, 2018).

The marketing of fortified pet foods and supplements closely resembles that of dietary supplements for humans. The same descriptors show up again and again: "natural," "clean," and "non-GMO" are favorites. Similar claims and assumptions are also made about what it takes to be well. Marketing campaigns position themselves not as salespeople but as "educators" who need to teach pet owners about their product's benefits, using language that sounds scientific and clinical but also emphasizes the supposed safety of relying on wholly "natural" cures. Sometimes the most effective sales tools seem at first to be an educational resource or website, but in truth they are sales platforms that exist for the purpose of pointing consumers to a particular product.

Dr. Freeman writes, "The pet food industry is a competitive one, with more and more companies joining the market every year. Marketing is a powerful tool for selling pet foods and has initiated and expanded fads." The prowess of marketers and the health-positioning of their product makes it difficult for pet owners to know what the best food for their pet truly is (as opposed to the one with the loudest or most attractive marketing). "Because of the thousands of diet choices, the creative and persuasive advertising, and the vocal opinions on the internet, pet owners aren't able to know if the diets they're feeding [their pets] have nutritional deficiencies or toxicities" (Freeman, 2018).

Let the buyer beware: avoid fads and be the skeptic. Most of the time, simply taking a walk is better for us than trying out the newest health trend. And that goes for dogs, too.

PET DIETARY SUPPLEMENTS: REGULATION, SAFETY, AND EFFICACY

So what about pet supplements specifically? So far, this chapter has dealt with the big picture of popular attitudes toward pet health and the pet industry's response in its product manufacturing and marketing. But what about my friend's question: Could a supplement be used to help an animal with aging issues or pain, or to combat a specific condition, such as arthritis?

If we looked only at the sales numbers for pet supplements, we would be tempted to say "yes." According to a report by Packaged Facts, "...factors related to COVID-19 caused sales of pet supplements to shoot up 21% in 2020 to nearly $800 million, quadrupling the rate of sales growth seen in 2019" (Packaged Facts, 2021). The most popular pet supplements are multivitamins, and the most popular condition-specific supplements are those that claim to promote joint or heart health, and to maintain coat and skin, followed by those that support the digestive tract (Burns, 2017). It is estimated that the sales of pet dietary supplements will exceed $1 billion by 2025 (Packaged Facts, 2021). For so many people to spend so much money, these products must have some efficacy, right?

Efficacy: The Science behind Pet Supplements

Unfortunately, there are few well-designed clinical trials on pet supplements to back up all these sales. Without knowing exactly what effect a supplement will have on the animal taking it, and what dosages are appropriate, the use of such supplements is inherently risky.

How can we sort through all the advertising and assess the usefulness of individual pet supplements? Organizations like the American Veterinary Medical Association are a good place to look for the latest developments in pet supplement science based on clinical trials involving the animals themselves.

What does science have to say, for instance, about one of the oldest and most common pet supplements, glucosamine?

Glucosamine, one of the components of cartilage, which cushions joints, has long been used to treat arthritis and joint pain. Though large human clinical trials have been conducted on glucosamine, the results were inconclusive and only mildly optimistic. This is one of the few areas in which many studies have also been conducted on dogs. But these trials were of varying quality, using different dosages, forms, and combinations of glucosamine products. Because the major objective is to alleviate pain, the results can also be difficult to quantify. All in all, researchers have not been able to show significant benefits (Bhathal et al., 2017).

In fact, in 2016, the American Veterinary Association issued a statement reversing its earlier endorsement of glucosamine. They claimed that it was not consistent with their "evidence-based" commitment. The science simply was not showing any convincing proof of its effectiveness. The good news is that these trials have shown that glucosamine in moderate doses is benign in its side effects. While not able to help much, it is unlikely to do much harm, either (Burns, 2017).

What about fish oil, which, after glucosamine, is the most common supplement added to a pet's diet?

The results of individual clinical studies have shown some hopeful signs that fish oil may be an effective anti-inflammatory intervention for dogs, especially when used in conjunction with other treatments such as glucosamine (Olivry et al., 2010). Fish oil may also treat the symptoms of arthritis, though with very marginal benefit. In one study of seventy-seven dogs with osteoarthritis, half were given fish oil supplements and the other half were given corn oil. After sixteen weeks, there was overall "not a major statistically significant benefit" found in the fish-oil group. The research team did find, however, "a true but small relief in symptoms" on some measures for the dogs taking fish oil, and they encouraged further study (Hielm-Bjorkman et al., 2012). But other trials have shown that both dogs and cats who take fish oil supplements can also experience harmful side effects, such as altered platelet function, which can result in bleeding, weight gain, and slow wound healing (Tudor, 2013).

Though there is significant interest in pet supplements and "functional" pet foods that are fortified with vitamins, minerals, and herbs, pet owners' concern about pet health is often better directed toward broader health practices. Under some circumstances, supplements may help an ill or malnourished pet, but for most pets on a standard scientifically formulated diet, deficiency is not the major health issue that they are facing: obesity is. In the United States, 56% of dogs are overweight or obese, as are 60% of cats (Association for Pet Obesity Prevention, 2018). Like people, the best way for overweight pets to become healthy and reduce stress on their bodies is not to take supplements, but to lose weight through exercise and portion control.

Regulation and Safety

Who is keeping track of the pet products that Americans are buying, and ensuring their safety?

The FDA has regulatory powers over pet supplements, which almost always fall into the same legal category as all other types of pet food and are treated as "animal feed." In addition, each state has its own standards and regulatory powers over animal feed determined by their Department of Agriculture.

Interestingly, the FDA and individual states take a backseat on creating regulatory guidelines. Instead, a private organization, the Association of American Feed Control Officials, establishes uniform labeling and quality standards for the industry, although it has no regulatory powers (Schlesinger & Day, 2017). Pet food companies themselves have always self-policed the industry to a certain extent, with the top producers forming trade associations that seek to standardize quality. In part, this is necessary because pet diets are so limited: Any pet diet must meet exactly all the nutritional requirements of the animals that they are intended for.

What many consumers do not know is that the FDA does not proactively monitor quality control for pet supplements on the front end. In practice, active FDA involvement will occur only after enough adverse effects have been reported, which may then force a recall of the product. This, as we know, is the same situation as for human dietary supplements. There is no mandated pre-market testing, and products are only investigated after enough reports are received of harm caused to consumers.

In 2007, for instance, the laissez-faire regulatory situation in the pet industry boiled over into one of the largest recalls in FDA history. A Chinese supplier of ingredients to multiple pet food manufacturers had tainted its wheat gluten with melamine to make it appear to have a higher protein level. Reports of kidney failure and pet death came from veterinarians and individuals across the country, and the frantic chase for an answer finally revealed the fraudulent supply chain. Over 5,000 different products were recalled under dozens of different labels and companies. The first company to suspect the problem, Menu Foods, alone, lost over $40 million dollars from the recall (FDA, 2018).

CONCLUSION (AND RECOMMENDATIONS)

First, it is common sense to check your pet's daily intake of nutrients before adding more nutrients to their diet. The American College of Veterinary Nutrition's website assures owners that "if your pet is eating a complete and balanced commercially available pet food, supplements are not recommended unless specifically prescribed by your veterinarian" (American College of Veterinary Nutrition, 2016). Do not let pressure from health-oriented marketing campaigns overwhelm your common sense.

Second, look for independent auditing of the company and product. It doesn't matter how chic, raw, expensive, professional, or homemade a supplement appears to be; the best way to know that it is not contaminated is to simply investigate each product. Check the FDA's website for recalls. And if you see a problem with a pet supplement, be sure to report it to the FDA's Consumer Complaints department through the portal available on their website (and listed below in the resource box).

Third, remember that supplements, including herbal remedies, may have adverse effects and/or interact with other medications or other supplements that your pet is taking (Lenox and Bauer, 2013). For example, if your pet is on any blood thinner medications, they should not take ginkgo biloba because the risk of bleeding increases. Excessive vitamin E can prevent blood from clotting around cuts and scratches, which can turn to profuse bleeding (Goodman & Trepanier, 2005). Though little testing has been done, it is likely that some supplements can decrease a pet's ability to absorb medication, just as with human beings.

In every case, adding a supplement or turning to a specialty diet for your pet should only be done with the recommendation and under the supervision of a veterinarian. Marketing is not a substitute for training and medical expertise.

And finally, keep in mind that the Amended Dietary Supplement Health and Education Act (1994) distinguished pet supplements from food additives and placed supplements in the same category as food. It also allowed supplement manufacturers to market and sell pet supplements without review—meaning the FDA is barred from regulating them. This means that you need to do your own research on the safety (and efficacy) of your pet supplements.

TAKEAWAYS

- According to the American College of Veterinary Nutrition: "If your pet is eating a complete and balanced commercially available pet food, supplements are not recommended unless specifically prescribed by your veterinarian."

- If your pet requires dietary supplements, investigate the manufacturer to make sure the supplement is of high quality.

- The dietary supplement that your pet is taking may cause adverse reactions or interact with prescription medications that your pet is taking.

ADDITIONAL RESOURCES

- Resources for reporting problems with pet supplements to the FDA.

  https://www.fda.gov/animal-veterinary/report-problem/how-report-pet-food-complaint

- Information on finding your state Feed Control Official.

  https://www.aafco.org/Regulatory

- Information regarding pet food safety recalls: American Veterinary Medical Association.

  https://www.avma.org/News/Issues/recalls-alerts/Pages/pet-food-safety-recalls-alerts-fullyear.aspx

- Resource for information regarding pet food nutrition: The Pet Food Institute.

  https://www.petfoodinstitute.org/

- Trade organization: The National Animal Supplement Council.

  https://nasc.cc/

- Information on veterinary nutrition: When Less is More: Sensible Use of Supplements. https://vetnutrition.tufts.edu/2018/11/sensible-use-of-supplements/

- Resources on how pet food is regulated.

  https://www.cnbc.com/2017/05/06/what-is-really-in-the-food-your-dog-or-cat-is-eating.html

  Book: One Nation Under Dog: America's Love Affair with Our Dogs, by Michael Schafer

REFERENCES

American College of Veterinary Nutrition. (2016). *Frequently asked questions*. American College of Veterinary Medicine. http://www.acvn.org/frequently-asked-questions/

American Pet Products Association. (2017). *Pet industry market size & ownership statistics*. American Pet Products Association. https://www.americanpetproducts.org/press_industrytrends.asp

Association for Pet Obesity Prevention. (2018, April 19). *2017 pet obesity survey results: U.S. pet obesity steadily increases, owners and veterinarians share views on pet food*. Association for Pet Obesity Prevention. https://petobesityprevention.org/2017/

Bhathal, A., Spryszak, M., Louizos, C., & Frankel, G. (2017). Glucosamine and chondroitin use in canines for osteoarthritis: A review. *Open Veterinary Journal, 7*(1), 36–49. doi: https://doi.org/10.4314/ovj.v7i1.6

Burns, K. (2017, January 4). *Assessing pet supplements*. American Veterinary Medical Association (AMVA). https://www.avma.org/News/JAVMANews/Pages/170115a.aspx

Food and Drug Administration. (2018, September 4). *Melamine pet food recall of 2007*. Department of Health and Human Services, Food and Drug Administration. https://www.fda.gov/animalveterinary/safetyhealth/recallswithdrawals/ucm129575.htm

Freeman, L.M. (2018, June 4). *A broken heart: Risk of heart disease in boutique or grain-free diets and exotic ingredients*. Cummings Veterinary Medical Center at Tufts University. http://vetnutrition.tufts.edu/2018/06/a-broken-heart-risk-of-heart-disease-in-boutique-or-grain-free-diets-and-exotic-ingredients/

Goodman, L., & Trepanier, L. (2005). *Potential drug interactions with dietary supplements*. Compendium on Continuing Education for the Practicing Veterinarian 27(10). Retrieved from: http://www.vetfolio.com/pharmacology/potential-drug-interactions-with-dietary-supplements

Hielm-Bjorkman A., Anturaniemi (o.s. Roine), J., Elo, K., Lappalainen, A.K., Junnila, J.J.T., & Laitinen-Vapaavouri, O.M. (2012). An un-commissioned randomized, placebo-controlled double-blind study to test the effect of deep-sea fish oil as a pain reliever for dogs suffering from canine OA. *BMC Veterinary Research, 8*(1), 157. https://bmcvetres.biomedcentral.com/articles/10.1186/1746-6148-8-157

Hoffman, J. (2018, July 24). Popular grain-free dog foods may be linked to heart disease. *The New York Times.* https://www.nytimes.com/2018/07/24/health/grain-free-dog-food-heart-disease.html

Kanakubo, K., Fascetti, A.J., & Larsen, J.A. (2015). Assessment of protein and amino acid concentrations and labeling adequacy of commercial vegetarian diets formulated for dogs and cats. *Journal of the American Veterinary Medical Association, 247*(4), 385–392. doi: https://doi.org/10.2460/javma.247.4.385

Lenox, C.E., & Bauer, J.E. (2013). Potential adverse effects of omega-3 fatty acids in dogs and cats. *Journal of Veterinary Internal Medicine/American College of Veterinary Internal Medicine, 27*(2), 217–26. https://onlinelibrary.wiley.com/doi/full/10.1111/jvim.12033. doi: https://doi.org/10.1111/jvim.12033

McDermott, M.T. (2017, June 6). The vegan dog. *The New York Times.* https://www.nytimes.com/2017/06/06/well/family/the-vegan-dog.html

National Animal Supplement Council. (2018, July 12). *FDA investigates potential link between diet, dog heart disease.* National Animal Supplement Council. https://nasc.cc/news/fda-investigates-link-between-dog-food-and-dcm/

Olivo, L. (2017). *Top quality nutrition for family pets.* Nutraceuticals World. https://www.nutraceuticalsworld.com/issues/2017-09/view_features/top-quality-nutrition-for-family-pets/.

Olivry, T., DeBoer, D.J., Favrot, C., Jackson, H.J., Mueller, R., Nuttall, T., & Prélaud, P. (2010). Treatment of canine atopic dermatitis: 2010 clinical practice guidelines from the international task force on canine atopic dermatitis. *Veterinary Dermatology, 21*(3), 233–48. https://www.researchgate.net/publication/281813708_Treatment

_of_canine_atopic_dermatitis_2015_updated_guidelines_from
_the_International_Committee_on_Allergic_Diseases_of_Animals
_ICADA. doi: https://doi.org/10.1111/j.1365-3164.2010.00889.x

Packaged Facts. (2021, January 20). *Pet supplements in the U.S., 8th ed.*
Packaged Facts.

Rogers, K. (2017, August 18). *Pet hotels are riding the booming market for animal luxuries.* CNBC: On the Money. https://www.cnbc.com/2017/08/18
/pet-hotels-are-riding-the-booming-market-for-animal-luxuries-.html

Schlesinger, J., & Day, A. (2017, May 6). *What is really in the food your dog or cat is eating?* CNBC: On the Money. https://www.cnbc.com/2017/05
/06/what-is-really-in-the-food-your-dog-or-cat-is-eating.html

Tesfom, G., and Birch, N.J. (2010). Do they buy for their dogs the way they buy for themselves? *Psychology and Marketing, 27*(9), 898–912. https://www.researchgate.net/publication/246866062_Do_They
_Buy_for_Their_Dogs_the_Way_They_Buy_for_Themselves. doi:
https://doi.org/10.1002/mar.20364

Tudor, K. (2013, August 8). *Fish oil: The dangers of too much.* Pet MD.
https://www.petmd.com/blogs/thedailyvet/ktudor/2013/aug/the
-dangers-of-too-much-fish-oil-30731

van Bree, F.P.J., Bokken, G.C.A.M., Mineur, R., Franssen, F., Opsteegh, M., van der Giessen, J.W.B., Lipman, L.J.A., & Overgaauw, P.A.M. (2018). Zoonotic bacteria and parasites found in raw meat-based diets for cats and dogs. *Veterinary Record, 182*(2), 50. https://
veterinaryrecord.bmj.com/content/182/2/50. doi: https://doi.org
/10.1136/vr.104535

CHAPTER 7

LEARNING HOW TO TAKE THE DIETARY SUPPLEMENTS YOU NEED

STORY

Over the past few years, I have sat down with many friends and family members and reviewed the dietary supplements they take. Time and again, a good question from an acquaintance or a talk with a friend has transformed into a free-of-charge "dietary supplement consultation" where we empty the contents of their medicine cabinets or a kitchen drawer onto a table. Each session takes about two hours, during which I ask them a series of questions that help create a full picture of their current health. I review any blood tests they have had performed and any physical symptoms that could indicate a potential deficiency, and I then carefully consider their over-the-counter and prescription medications to check for potential negative interactions with their dietary supplements.

What are the results of these sessions? On average, I set aside about half (or more) of the dietary supplements that are part of their daily regimen, either because they do not need them or because the supplements could interact with their medications and potentially result in harmful supplement-drug interactions.

Then I look at the supplements that made the cut and investigate the company that manufactured the particular brand my friend or family member is taking. To do this, I first look for the stamps of official third-party companies that had verified the quality of that particular supplement. I say official because many "verified" or "approved" or "quality guaranteed" stamps that you will see on the bottles are meaningless (more on this later). Then I get my laptop and go on to the internet to learn about the company's record. Sometimes the supplement manufacturer does not pass my quality test. On a few occasions, I have even discovered that the FDA has issued recalls, injunctions, or seizure letters to the manufacturers of these products. By the time we are done with our review, there can be a small mountain of discarded supplements that were not needed, were of low quality, or were even unsafe. I ask my friends to dispose of their dietary supplements in the same manner that they would dispose of their expired or unused prescription medications, by finding an authorized collector in their community (see the contact information in the Additional Resources box).

At the beginning of these consultations, I ask everyone the same question: "Why do you take these supplements?" The answers are always as colorful as the bottles of the dietary supplements themselves. One friend told me, "I take them because Dr. Oz recommended them." I asked her if she had met with Dr. Oz, and if he had recommended them based on reviewing her blood tests and symptoms. The answer, of course, was no: "He recommended them on TV!"

Another friend told me that her naturopathic doctor recommended that she take the herbal supplement ginkgo biloba to improve her memory. The same friend was already taking the prescription drug warfarin (the generic name for Coumadin®) because she has had a mitral valve replacement in her heart. She forgot to tell her naturopathic doctor that she was taking warfarin, and she had no idea that ginkgo could negatively interact with warfarin and make her bleed. I could go on and on, sharing many more stories, but I think the point is clear. Exotic or seemingly urbane supplements taken without consideration of your body's actual needs, or without any knowledge of the quality of the product, can be harmful. The purpose of this chapter is to teach you how to ask the right questions that will lead you to the right dietary supplements for you.

ASK THE RIGHT QUESTIONS TO GET THE RIGHT ANSWERS

Before taking any dietary supplements, you need to ask yourself a very basic question: "Do I need this supplement?" A good healthcare provider can help you find the answer, but you also need to know what to ask for and how to be your own advocate.

Ask for the Right Blood Test

First, ask for a standard blood test that checks your nutritional status and assesses the functions of your organs (e.g., liver, kidney, heart, thyroid). The blood test should evaluate your electrolytes (including calcium, magnesium, and phosphorous) and include a metabolic panel that includes fasting glucose, creatinine, liver function tests, vitamin D levels, folate and homocysteine levels, DHA/EPA, and a lipid panel.

This is the most helpful starting place to screen your body for deficiencies. Your blood is a microcosm of your whole body, and a regular blood test can detect many vitamin and mineral deficiencies. For hospital patients in critical condition, the standard procedure is to perform blood tests frequently in order to monitor their vitamin, mineral, and electrolyte levels, and then carefully replenish the body with what it needs through intravenous nutrition. Blood tests are invaluable and essential—the obvious first step for anyone who might have a vitamin or mineral deficiency.

But sometimes a standard blood test is not sufficient, and you may need a more elaborate one (e.g., if you need a more comprehensive assessment of your nutritional status). Several tests on the market claim to provide you with a comprehensive analysis of your nutritional status. These tests might analyze your hair, saliva, urine, blood, and even DNA, but for the most part there is no research to support these tests as reliable methods to determine which dietary supplements you need. Except for a few minor mutations, our DNA does not change as we age. We have the same DNA that we were born with, and it is therefore not the most helpful place to look to assess nutrition. When it comes to blood, urine, saliva, or hair testing, these tests have innate limitations in the degree to which they can comprehensively and accurately analyze your nutritional status. For instance, some essential elements and vitamins circulate in your blood while others are stored in fat tissues or organs and are then released in your systemic circulation (blood) when needed, so they are not all equally observable. Furthermore, these tests are more like snapshots; they reflect your nutritional status based on what you recently ate and your activities during a short period before you had the tests. To get an accurate assessment of your actual nutritional status, you would need to repeat these tests on different days at different times. But this approach is time-consuming and expensive. Though blood tests also have their limitations, consider doing a basic but comprehensive assessment of your nutritional status on a day during a week that represents a typical day and week in your life.

For this purpose, various blood tests can be performed. Many of these tests are sold online directly to consumers with prices ranging from $99 to $999 and from testing techniques ranging from at-home point-of-care to venipuncture (drawing blood from a vein). I reviewed the scientific literature to see if I could find any published studies on the quality or validity of these tests. I was not able to find large outcome studies on the value that these tests may add to overall health, but I found small validation studies comparing an isolated blood bio-marker measured in a point-of-care test to that measured in a regular venipuncture test. If you have health insurance, you may be able to get these tests covered if your doctor orders them. To be reimbursed, sometimes the doctor must request the tests to investigate a particular problem or symptom rather than as part of a "checkup."

Regardless of who orders and performs your blood test, you need to share them with a healthcare provider. Your healthcare provider should combine the results of these tests with your other health and personal data, such as lifestyle, family history, diet, symptoms, illnesses, and medications, to come up with an assessment of your nutritional status and deficiencies in vitamins, minerals, enzymes, etc.

However, when you receive your results, you also need to remember that low levels of a nutrient (not overt deficiencies) are in some cases very relative. People may have a wide variation of levels and still be healthy. If you are slightly low in a vitamin or mineral, my recommendation is to try to modify your diet to manage the deficiency rather than taking a dietary supplement and repeat the test in a few months.

What Can a Blood Test Show?

Especially when people age, facing new life stages and physical challenges, their bodies may not absorb nutrients as well as they once did, even if their diet is a healthy one. In some cases, a blood test can quickly catch these problems.

For example, an easily identified problem is vitamin deficiency anemia. This is indicated on a blood test when the red blood cell count is low. If, for example, the deficiency is in vitamin B12 or folate, the red blood cell count (often reported as the "hematocrit," the percentage of blood volume made up by red cells) will be low, and the cells themselves are also "large and underdeveloped" (Mayo Foundation for Medical Education and Research, 2018a). Because red blood cells move oxygen throughout the body, vitamin deficiency anemia forces your body to work much harder to get the oxygen it needs. The initial physical symptoms for vitamin B12–deficiency anemia are fatigue and weakness; the chances for this kind of deficiency increase as you age, if you have cancer, and for pregnant women. Vitamin B12 deficiency, if severe and prolonged, can also cause nerve and spinal cord damage. Fortunately, once diagnosed, it is easily treated with vitamin B12 supplementation.

Blood tests are one of the most valuable ways to read what is happening in your body. However, while blood tests have long been used to test for certain kinds of deficiencies, these tests have major limitations that you should be aware of. Any type of blood test should be interpreted by a healthcare provider with expertise in nutritional assessment.

HOW TO INTERPRET AND ACT
UPON BLOOD TEST RESULTS

Blood tests require interpretation. They need to be carefully reviewed and the results weighed against the existing scientific consensus. In some cases, the "right" blood level of a nutrient is unknown, or the normal range can vary greatly from person to person without seeming to cause any harm. And some deficiencies are more difficult to reliably trace than others. In this section, I will give some specific examples of how blood tests can be used to inform dietary supplementation.

Folate

Folate is a water-soluble member of the B-vitamin family that plays an important role in metabolism. Folate is present in numerous foods, particularly green leafy vegetables, and since 1998 has been added to flours and cereals in the U.S. Normal blood folate levels are >3 ng/mL. Because of the abundance of dietary sources, folate deficiency is rare and usually limited to those with poor diet (e.g., alcoholics) or people suffering from malabsorption. Blood folate levels rapidly normalize upon eating a normal diet, so the amount of folate present within red blood cells, which last 120 days in the circulation, can be a better long-term measure of folate intake. The Recommended Dietary Allowance (RDA) of folate is 400 micrograms (mcg) in adults. As discussed above, folate deficiency causes anemia and is associated with fetal neural tube defects in pregnant women. Folate deficiency has also been postulated to increase the risk of depression, dementia, and some forms of cancer, although definitive evidence is lacking.

Should you take folate supplements? If you are healthy and eat a balanced diet, it is pretty unlikely that you are folate deficient. There is no evidence that ingestion of more than the RDA of folate will be beneficial, and actually there is some concern that taking more than 1,000 mcg daily might have deleterious effects on the immune system from unmetabolized folic acid (Troen et al., 2006).

In its role in cellular metabolism, folate is processed by a series of enzymes, including one called methylene tetrahydrofolate reductase or MTHFR for short. Some individuals (including 25% of Hispanics and 10% of Caucasians and Asians) have inherited a mutation in the gene for MTHFR that causes reduced activity. This results in a metabolic condition that is similar to folate deficiency, although folate levels are normal. One consequence is an increase in homocysteine levels, which is a risk factor for cardiovascular disease. Individuals with elevated homocysteine levels may benefit from supplementation with the "active" form of folate, l-5-methyltetrahydrofolate or 5-MHTF (Akoglu et al., 2008).

Vitamin B12

As mentioned above, proper levels of vitamin B12 are essential for the health of your blood and neurological systems. B12 is naturally present in animal products but not plants, although most cereals are B12-fortified. For a person with a healthy diet and normal food absorption, vitamin B12 deficiency is very uncommon. People at risk for B12 deficiency include strict vegetarians and those with gastrointestinal disorders or who have had gastrointestinal surgery. The blood level of vitamin B12 is readily measured, and levels below 170–250 pg/mL may be indicative of deficiency. However, there is some evidence that blood concentrations of B12 may not reflect that in the tissues, and your doctor can also check the level of methylmalonic acid (MMA), which, if elevated, can indicate a metabolic response to borderline levels of vitamin B12, confirming a deficiency. Ironically, supplementation with folate can mask the effect of B12 deficiency on the blood system, preventing anemia but not the neurological damage.

The RDA of vitamin B12 is 2.4 mcg for adults (a bit higher for pregnant or nursing females) and can be supplemented by mouth, with the exception of patients with a condition known as pernicious anemia.

Pernicious anemia is an autoimmune disorder occurring most commonly in individuals of northern European ancestry where the stomach lining is affected, causing deficiency of a protein (intrinsic factor) that is necessary for the efficient absorption of vitamin B12 from the intestine. Left untreated, these individuals will eventually develop B12 deficiency and suffer from anemia and neurologic disease. It is important to recognize malabsorption of B12 as the underlying cause of the deficiency, because this condition should be treated by B12 injections rather than by the oral route. B12 malabsorption can be diagnosed by one of several laboratory tests ordered by a doctor.

Vitamin D

Vitamin D deficiency is often cited as the most common nutrient deficiency in the United States. In recent years, as vitamin D deficiency has gained more attention, blood tests to diagnose this problem have been on the rise. At face value, this seems like a good thing. Surely, if more people know they are low in vitamin D, they can use supplements and live healthier lives, right?

A challenge with blood tests is the common misperception of what it takes to "fix" a deficiency. Many nutrition experts are concerned that people woefully oversimplify what a deficiency means. The health problems associated with low vitamin D levels, for instance, may not be strictly caused by too little intake of the nutrient, but rather from an unhealthy lifestyle that generally accompanies low D levels. Since vitamin D is made by our bodies when we are exposed to sunlight, people with low levels of vitamin D may be overweight and spend little time exercising and outside; vitamin D deficiency is sometimes a symptom of a larger problem, rather than the problem itself.

Another difficulty is that currently there is no agreement in the medical community about what level of vitamin D is "too low"; different practitioners may follow different guidelines. And, to make matters murkier, the tests used for measuring vitamin D levels vary. The form of vitamin D that should be measured is called 25-hydroxyvitamin D or 25(OH)D. Blood levels of the active form of vitamin D, 1,25$(OH)_2$D, are too variable and unreliable. So, what should your 25(OH)D level be? The Food and Nutrition Board (FNB) of the National Academies of Science, Engineering, and Medicine concluded that people with 25(OH)D levels below 12 ng/mL are at risk for vitamin D deficiency (Institute of Medicine, 2010). In contrast, the Endocrine Society (an international group of endocrine and metabolism professionals) considers a level ≥ 20 ng/mL as adequate for bone and overall health in healthy individuals (Holick et al., 2011). The NIH ODS website has an excellent "Fact Sheet for Consumers" about vitamin D with a discussion about these issues (NIH ODS, 2020).

Should you be tested for vitamin D levels and take vitamin D supplements? Vitamin D testing is quite common in the United States, often done annually as part of a routine health checkup. In spite of this, the U.S. Preventive Services Task Force concludes, "The current evidence is insufficient to assess the balance of benefits and harms of screening for vitamin D deficiency in asymptomatic adults" (United States Preventive Services Task Force, 2021). For people with 25(OH)D levels below 20 ng/mL, vitamin D supplementation is recommended. A reasonable goal for healthy individuals is to keep your 25(OH)D between 20 and 50 ng/mL, as the FNB noted that levels > 50 ng/mL can be associated with adverse effects.

What is the evidence that vitamin D supplementation in healthy people can help prevent or treat medical conditions such as osteoporosis, cancer, cardiovascular disease, autoimmune disease, or infections? Unfortunately, there is little research that supports the use of vitamin D supplements in these scenarios. For osteoporosis, the United States Preventive Services Task Force has concluded that "...daily supplementation with 400 IU or less of vitamin D and 1000 mg or less of calcium has no benefit for the primary prevention of fractures in community-dwelling, postmenopausal women," and that there is "inadequate evidence to estimate the benefits of doses greater than 400 IU of vitamin D or greater than 1000 mg of calcium to prevent fractures" for such women (United States Preventive Services Task Force, 2018). In 2019, a very large U.S. study on vitamin D3 (or cholecalciferol) was completed using 25,871 participants, all of whom were men over fifty and women over fifty-five. The study was randomized and controlled—meaning that there was one group taking vitamin D3 along with an omega-3 fatty acid (to aid absorption) and another group who was taking a placebo. The findings showed that the supplemented group did not have a lower incidence of invasive cancers—breast, prostate, or colorectal—nor was there any reduction in cardiovascular problems (Manson et al., 2019). For information about vitamin D and COVID-19 infection, please see the appendix.

In summary, based on the current scientific literature, we should take vitamin D only if we have vitamin D deficiency. A reasonable recommendation is that if 25(OH)D levels are below 20 ng/mL (50 nmol/L) then supplementation is warranted. But as of now, there is no causal association between vitamin D levels in the range above this level and the prevention of disease.

Of course, as always, you should consult with your healthcare provider to decide whether or not you need vitamin D supplementation. Some genetic predispositions may cause your optimal vitamin D levels to be different than the above recommendation.

Iron

Iron is an essential component of hemoglobin, the protein in red blood cells that carries oxygen (and makes them red!), myoglobin in your muscles, and several other important cellular enzymes. Your body normally contains about 3–4 grams of iron in several different forms. The majority of the iron is in red cells, while most of the rest is in a storage form in the liver, spleen, and bone marrow, complexed with a protein called ferritin. Everyone loses small amounts of iron every day by shedding of cells in the gastrointestinal tract, and this is replaced by iron from the diet. However, females are at risk for losing more iron because of menstrual bleeding and pregnancy.

Your body closely regulates iron levels by monitoring the amount of iron in your blood, which is bound to a transport protein called transferrin. When the level of transferrin-bound iron falls, the body attempts to compensate by absorbing more iron from the GI tract and liberating iron from stores. Hence, the first signs of iron deficiency that can be detected on a blood test are a low percentage of iron-bound transferrin (normally 15–50%) and low serum ferritin (normally 20–250 ng/mL). If the condition persists, the deficiency of iron will begin to affect the production of new red blood cells in the bone marrow, leading to a form of anemia where the red cells are small and pale. Besides fatigue, symptoms of iron deficiency include impaired cognitive and immune function. These can be particularly severe in children, leading to prolonged learning difficulties. The prevalence of iron deficiency in the population varies by socioeconomic and racial/ethnic status: in the U.S., 6% of Caucasian and Black children aged 1–3 have iron deficiency compared with 12% of Hispanic children (Brotanek et al., 2007). Similarly, among pregnant women, 24–30% of Black and Hispanic females are iron-deficient compared with 14% of non-Hispanic Whites (Mei et al., 2011).

Based on the above statistics, screening for iron deficiency, particularly in women and young children, is warranted. The important blood tests are transferrin saturation and ferritin levels. For ferritin, one caveat is that inflammation can cause elevations in ferritin that are not reflective of iron stores, so care is needed in interpreting ferritin levels in the low-normal range. How can we prevent and treat iron deficiency? Again, the best approach is through the diet. The RDA for iron is 8–11 mg for growing children, 8 mg for adult men, and 18 mg for adult women (27 mg for pregnant women and 8 mg for post-menopausal women). Iron is present in many natural foods, including lean meat, seafood, poultry, beans, peas, and lentils, and is also added to some fortified food products such as cereal. The iron in lean meat and seafood is in the form of heme (bound to a chemical scaffold from hemoglobin or myoglobin) and is efficiently absorbed from the GI tract. By contrast, the non-heme form of iron in plants is less well-absorbed and some plants also contain substances (polyphenols) that interfere with iron absorption. This can be partly overcome by taking vitamin C, which promotes iron absorption.

While most people obtain adequate iron from their diet, this may not be the case for infants, young children, teenage girls, pregnant women, and premenopausal women. For them, there are a wide variety of iron supplements available. Small amounts of iron (10–18 mg) are present in many multivitamin products. There are also iron-only supplements providing larger amounts (45–65 mg) of iron complexed with different chemicals, including sulfate, gluconate, and citrate. These different forms of iron contain varying amounts of actual iron. For example, ferrous sulfate is 20% iron while ferrous gluconate is 12%, so it is important to check the label of your supplement. The major side effect of taking iron supplements is constipation, which can be minimized by starting slowly (half a tablet a day, or every other day) and by eating plenty of fiber. Rarely, someone with gastrointestinal disease or surgery may not absorb oral iron, in which case the doctor can prescribe intravenous iron supplements. Iron supplements can also interact or interfere with several medications, including the drug levodopa in Parkinson's disease patients and levothyroxine in patients with thyroid deficiency. Check with your doctor before taking iron supplements if you have these conditions.

It is also possible to get too much iron! When ferritin levels exceed 250 ng/mL or transferrin saturation approaches 90%, there can be free iron in the circulation that can damage the heart, liver, and pancreas. Iron overload can be seen in patients who have had frequent blood transfusions, certain blood disorders, and in a rare inherited condition called hemochromatosis. There is little risk that a healthy adult with normal intestinal function will develop iron overload, but most older men and postmenopausal women probably do not need supplemental iron. The risks of accidental iron overdose in children are discussed below.

Fish Oil Supplements

Fish and fish products are rich in omega-3 fatty acids, including docosahexaenoic acid (DHA) and eicosapentaenoic acid (EHA). Many studies have shown that people who eat fatty fish and other seafood have a lower risk of several chronic diseases, including heart disease, cancer, and dementia. However, it is not clear whether there is a cause-and-effect relationship between intake of these foods or of omega-3 fatty acids and these health outcomes, and more research including RCTs is needed. There are several methods to check the levels of omega-3s in your blood. One is the omega-3 index, which measures the relative amount of DHA and EPA in the membranes of your red blood cells and is expressed as a percent (> 8% is considered optimal). It is also possible to measure DHA and EPA levels directly, although there is less confidence about what represents an optimal level.

There are several meta-analysis studies that suggest a correlation between omega-3 levels and coronary heart disease (Del Gobbo et al., 2016), which may in part be due to lowering of triglyceride levels. For patients with coronary heart disease (CHD), omega-3 supplementation seems to reduce the risk of heart attack and death (Hu et al., 2019) and the EPA supplement icosapent ethyl (Vascepa®) received FDA approval in 2019 for patients with CHD and high triglyceride levels (Boden et al., 2020). Similarly, some but not all observational studies have suggested that omega-3 intake is associated with a decreased risk of cognitive impairment or dementia. While clinical trials show no effect of omega-3 supplementation on patients with established Alzheimer's disease, there may be improvements in patients with mild cognitive defects (Mazereeuw et al., 2012). Unfortunately, there is little evidence to suggest a role for omega-3 levels or supplementation on cancer, eye disease, depression, or inflammatory bowel disease, although studies in these and many other conditions are ongoing.

Should you take fish oil supplements? If you have a serious medical condition, particularly coronary heart disease, you should consult with your doctor. For otherwise healthy adults, it would be reasonable to check your omega-3 index. If it is low, reassess your diet and see if increasing the amount of fish and other seafood is realistic. Consumption of about eight ounces per week of a variety of seafood, which provides an average consumption of 250 mg per day of EPA and DHA, is recommended. Make sure to choose fish that are low in methylmercury content (i.e., avoid predator fish like tuna, marlin, and swordfish). If supplements are contemplated, it is important to consider both the source of the supplement (as discussed elsewhere) and the dose. For patients with CHD, the American Heart Association recommends approximately 1 g per day of total EPA/DHA. The FDA's approach to fish oil supplements has evolved over the years. In 2004, the agency approved a qualified health claim for foods and supplements that contain EPA and DHA that stated, "Supportive but not conclusive research shows that consumption of EPA and DHA omega-3 fatty acids may reduce the risk of coronary heart disease." Subsequently, in June 2019, the FDA approved the use by supplement manufacturers of qualified health claims that consuming EPA and DHA may reduce the risk of hypertension and CHD (FDA, 2019). Dietary supplements bearing such a claim must contain at least 0.8 g of combined EPA and DHA per serving. So how much fish oil supplement should you take? A study of the relationship between omega-3 dose and the effect on the omega-3 index showed that this is affected by body weight, age, and sex. Depending on your baseline omega-3 index, this information can help you decide how much omega-3s you might consider taking. For example, an omega-3 dose of 900 mg daily leads to a 75% increase in the omega-3 index (Flock et al., 2013).

Trace Elements

There are many chemicals, including manganese, copper, zinc, molybdenum, selenium, and chromium (the so-called "trace elements") that have important functions in the body, usually by helping different enzymes function properly. Deficiencies in these elements can cause symptoms (National Research Council, 1989). Many of these deficiency states were discovered in patients receiving all their nutrition by the intravenous route (so-called total parenteral nutrition), where it became necessary to add these elements to the nutrition solution. Blood levels of these elements may not reflect total body stores and are not routinely measured. As mentioned above, there are many places that offer analysis of hair or saliva to assess levels of these trace elements. However, the role of hair analysis in the diagnosis and management of trace element deficiency has not been clearly established. RDAs for these elements have been defined, and trace element deficiency in healthy people with normal diet and intestinal function is extremely uncommon (Institute of Medicine, 2001). Most multivitamin supplements contain amounts of trace elements ranging from 30–200% of the respective RDAs. The NIH ODS website has very informative fact sheets on most of the trace elements (https://ods.od.nih.gov/factsheets/list-all/).

DO YOUR HOMEWORK

Many people fall into the temptation of thinking a deficiency is something that can be easily fixed with supplements rather than as a signal to ask important questions about their overall health. My recommendation is to find a healthcare provider who can help you accurately assess your blood tests, as well as your overall lifestyle and nutritional status, and then guide you to practices that will truly improve your health.

Ask About the Dietary Supplement Manufacturers

If you do need dietary supplements, remember that these products' quality and trustworthiness vary greatly. Unlike pharmaceuticals, supplements are available to consumers without undergoing rigorous pre-market testing. Contamination and fraudulent labeling are common and usually caught only once they cause harm. Recently, Consumer Lab tested fifty different multivitamins and found problems with 46% of the tested products. Twelve contained different amounts of the vitamins than what was listed on the label, many had far more of different substances than is recommended for daily intake, and some failed in absorption tests (Cooperman, 2020). Ask your healthcare provider about how to choose the best possible supplement (not the most expensive, but the highest quality) and to verify the correct dosage for you. I personally believe that the provider should not have any financial conflict of interest with the supplement manufacturer that they recommend. In other words, you should not be buying supplements directly from your healthcare provider. If they do sell the recommended supplements, they should disclose any potential conflict of interest clearly.

Once you have a professional recommendation, do a little fact-checking on your own. In chapter 3, I walked you through my recommendations for how to locate quality producers. I will review the highlights here.

How Do You Find a Trustworthy Dietary Supplement Manufacturer?

Look for a company that follows the good manufacturing practices set by the FDA. These companies often have the U.S. Pharmacopeia (USP) stamp on their products. The U.S. Pharmacopeia verification process includes assessing the manufacturing process, the product's quality, the sources of its ingredients, and its bioavailability. U.S. Pharmacopeia evaluates the dietary supplement one to six times per year using samples purchased in stores as opposed to samples provided by the company. Thoughtful companies should be making all of this information easily available to their customers, providing websites that link to reports that showcase the independent testing of their products.

Check the FDA website. All you need to do is type in the name of the product or its manufacturer to see if they are being investigated. All the warning letters the FDA has sent to these companies are readily available for the public to see, as are any FDA recalls of products.

Any dietary supplement can be contaminated if not handled properly, but many FDA recalls are the result of the purposeful adulteration of dietary supplements with drugs, to make them more effective. Weight-loss, sports enhancement, and sexual enhancement supplements are the top targets for adulteration. According to a published FDA list of tainted dietary supplements, 37% of the 416 public alerts that were launched between 2010 and 2015 corresponded to adulterated natural weight-loss products (Rocha et al., 2015). These "all-natural" weight-loss aids were spiked with substances such as sibutramine, a dieting drug pulled off the U.S. market in 2010 because it caused enhanced risk of stroke and cardiovascular problems. Phenolpthalein, a laxative that some studies have linked to cancer, has also been found by the FDA to be illegally added to some weight-loss products. But the most frequent recalls are for sexual enhancement supplements. Also from 2010 to 2015, the FDA issued 229 public notifications for sexual enhancement dietary supplements. These alerts represented more than half of all public notifications regarding dietary supplements during this time period. What was hidden in these products? Viagra or other prescription drugs for erectile dysfunction were mixed in, creating "a very high risk to consumers' health" (Rocha et al., 2015). Again, information about these recalls are always publicly available through the FDA recall portal.

Another helpful consumer advocacy group to check before you make a purchase is Consumer Lab (www.consumerlab.com). While they do not conduct scientific testing in the same way as U.S.

Pharmacopeia, they are an independent organization that checks for the relative quality of similar products.

Monitor the Dietary Supplement's Efficacy

Once you begin taking a supplement, your healthcare provider (and you) should monitor your progress to make sure the supplement works and that it is safe for you. This is what should happen any time you take something that has a pharmacological effect, whether it be prescription drugs, over-the-counter medications, or dietary supplements.

Schedule a follow-up appointment. How is your body reacting one month later? Ask your provider when it would make sense to have another blood test performed to check on your body's absorption of the supplement and to make sure that the supplement is not causing any health issues.

Supplements may serve a purpose, but they are not a magic bullet or a quick fix for all physical problems. The automatic solution for a deficiency is not always a dietary supplement; changes in diet may be the better way to get exactly what your body needs. It is also possible that the deficiency is a signal that your body has an underlying problem that needs to be addressed, and further evaluation and tests may be necessary. Throughout this process, having a conscientious and well-informed healthcare provider is vital, but you also need to act as your own advocate and try to be as informed as you can.

A good conversation about supplements should be part of a broader discussion about what will make your life healthier and happier.

How Can You Monitor for the Safety of the Supplements You Take?

"First, do no harm"—this fundamental rule of medicine has guided physicians for centuries, and should be our goal as well. Dietary supplements can be potent. If they have the ability to help us and result in physiological changes in our bodies, that means they can harm us if taken in the wrong way or in an inappropriate dosage. One of the fundamental motivations for me to write this book was to challenge the misconception that, because supplements are "natural," they are always safe. Here are the three safety concerns that I would advise everyone who takes supplements to be aware of:

Toxicity

Each year, almost 60,000 cases of vitamin toxicity are reported to U.S. poison-control centers (Rosenbloom, 2020). A study funded by the U.S. HHS that was published in 2015 estimated that annually 23,000 emergency department visits in the United States are attributed to adverse events from dietary supplements. Among the most reported adverse events were cardiovascular symptoms from weight-loss or energy products among young adults, and swallowing problems, often associated with micronutrients, among older adults (Geller et al., 2015).

In excessive amounts, or in the wrong combination, supplements can become toxic. The risk of toxicity is lower with water-soluble vitamins, but higher with those vitamins that are fat-soluble—especially vitamins A, D, E, and K. Since your body is not able to easily process and get rid of excess fat-soluble vitamins, these vitamins get stored in fat tissues for long periods of time and eventually are released back into the body.

Long-term intake of vitamin A, for instance, can lead to carotenemia, which is not dangerous, but causes yellow pigmentation of the skin. Vitamins containing iron are especially risky. The body cannot process excess iron, and the excess iron can corrode the lining of the stomach and digestive tract. During the 1980s, the third leading cause of poisoning in children resulting in death was from overconsumption of iron, especially the kind made in the form of adult supplements that looked like candy. Fortunately, laws requiring warning labels on high-iron supplements and childproof caps, as well as other reforms in the industry (no longer coating iron tablets in sugar), have made iron poisoning in children less common over the past twenty years (National Institutes of Health, 2018). Taking excessive amounts of vitamin D can also be dangerous. The RDA of vitamin D for most adults is 600 international units (IU) per day. While up to 4,000 IU daily is probably safe, taking higher doses can lead to elevations in blood calcium levels, causing nausea and vomiting, dehydration, and possibly kidney stones (Zeratsky, 2020). Fish oil supplements containing large amounts of omega-3 fatty acids can cause decreased function of blood platelets and an increased tendency for bleeding.

Be vigilant about doses. If you are taking multiple supplements, check carefully that you are not accidentally doubling up on your intake.

And finally, make sure to have a baseline blood test prior to taking any supplements (or pharmaceuticals). Dietary supplements can cause organ damage (e.g., kidney and liver). A very close friend developed major liver toxicity, ironically, after being on a "liver detox" program that contained a variety of dietary supplements (including herbs) for three months. Prior to being on this program, she had seen her regular physician, who had ordered a complete blood test for her. Her liver function tests (AST and ALT, which if elevated can indicate liver injury) were normal at that time. (I am not sure why she even thought that she needed to "detox" her liver!) After following the liver detox program for three months, her liver enzymes tests showed a dangerous 100-fold increase. If she had continued taking those dietary supplements, she might have required a liver transplant!

Supplement-Drug and Supplement-Supplement Interactions

Almost 25% of U.S. adults take prescription medication and dietary supplements at the same time—and most do not tell their physicians that they are taking supplements (Asher et al., 2017). In

THE TRUTH ABOUT DIETARY SUPPLEMENTS

the wrong combination, dietary supplements can interact with medications and either inhibit their effectiveness or dangerously enhance them.

Warfarin (Coumadin®), a drug used to treat and prevent blood clots, can have disastrous interactions with common supplements and should not be taken with garlic extract, St. John's wort, green tea, ginseng, vitamin E, or coenzyme Q10 (Mayo Foundation for Medical Education and Research, 2018b). St. John's wort, a commonly used supplement for anxiety and depression, for example, can speed up the time that it takes your body to break down (metabolize) certain medications, which can inhibit the effectiveness of a drug like warfarin. St. John's wort has also been shown to reduce the effectiveness of some birth control pills and HIV/AIDS drugs (Gardiner et al., 2008).

Sometimes supplements and drugs perform similar functions, which means that taking them both at once would have the same effect as an overdose. This is true of supplements that affect serotonin levels. If St. John's wort is taken with antidepressants like paroxetine (Paxil®), fluoxetine (Prozac®), or any drug that increases serotonin levels, serotonin syndrome can be precipitated. When too much serotonin builds up in a person's system, dizziness, heart palpitations, and in extreme cases, unconsciousness and death can follow.

In addition to supplement-drug interactions, supplements can adversely interact with each other. For instance, vitamin E, while not toxic itself in moderate amounts, can block the effect of vitamin K, which in turn can cause coagulopathy, or the inability of the blood to clot enough to prevent bleeding (Rosenbloom, 2020).

These adverse reactions can be mild or severe, but any harm done is all the more problematic because most people are not on the alert for any symptoms. We are conditioned to watch for the risks associated with prescription drugs or even the most common over-the-counter medications, such as cough syrup, but unfortunately, we are not taught to treat dietary supplements with the same care.

Make sure that your healthcare provider knows which supplements you are taking and can help you avoid an accidental adverse reaction. If you see multiple healthcare providers, make sure to share a list of all your prescription drugs and dietary supplements with all of them.

Hidden Risks: Supplements Interfering with Blood Lab Results

In November 2017, the FDA put out an official warning concerning vitamin B7, or biotin. The report alerted "the public, healthcare providers, lab personnel, and lab test developers that biotin can significantly interfere with certain lab tests and cause incorrect test results which may go undetected" (FDA, 2017). Biotin can skew blood results and make them appear to be artificially high or low, making it easy to misdiagnose a patient during a crisis. The FDA warns specifically about its ability to mask troponin levels, which is a key indicator of heart muscle damage. Because vitamin B7 or biotin is often added to beauty and health products that claim to boost hair and nail health, it is possible for people to be taking excessive amounts of biotin without knowing it.

CONCLUSION

Supplements may or may not be part of what you need for optimum health. Make these decisions based on the best science available and your body's actual needs, rather than on the deafening noise of supplement marketing that hopes to sell you as many products as possible. Pursue this path with a trustworthy and skilled healthcare provider. Each year, thousands of unnecessary life-threatening episodes of toxicity and adverse interactions occur that could have been prevented. Don't blindly experiment on yourself. Instead, become informed so that you can ask the best questions possible and know where to look for the most trustworthy sources of information. And, because your body and its needs will change over time, take the long view. Pay attention to your body and your symptoms, repeat blood tests, and when appropriate, reassess the supplements that you take.

TAKEAWAYS

- A supplement may have been beneficial for a friend or a celebrity, but that does not mean that it is good for everyone. Take supplements and your own body's needs seriously. Do not take supplements based on attractive marketing or anecdotes.

- To learn if there are any supplements that you should take, visit a healthcare provider and get an overall assessment of your current health and any medications you are on or special conditions to consider. Then, request a blood test that maps your general state of health and nutritional needs.

- Blood tests are not perfect, but they are the simplest way to check for an obvious deficiency.

- Know that there is a wide range of healthy levels for many minerals and nutrients, and that for some substances, the jury is still out on what an appropriate level is.

- If, after a full checkup and a blood test, you and your healthcare provider decide a supplement is needed, choose a high-quality supplement from a manufacturer whose products have been certified by a trustworthy independent regulatory board such as USP.

- Below are the logos of two of the companies, U.S. Pharmacopeia and NSF International, that assure a better quality for that dietary supplement.

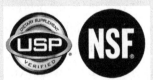

- Finally, follow up. Monitor how you are feeling, and go back for a follow-up blood test to make sure that the supplement you are on is safe and effective.

- Recognize that your body and its needs change. Something you need now may not be appropriate five or ten years from now, and vice versa.

ADDITIONAL RESOURCES

- Resources on drug-supplement (and drug-drug) interactions.

  https://www.webmd.com/interaction-checker/default.htm

- Information regarding potential FDA investigations of manufacturers of dietary supplements.

  https://www.fda.gov/

- Database of all FDA-approved home and lab tests for blood tests.

  https://www.accessdata.fda.gov/scripts/cdrh/cfdocs/cfIVD/Search.cfm

- Resources regarding the proper disposal of unwanted dietary supplements (and prescription drugs): Drug Enforcement Administration.

  https://www.dea.gov

  National Prescription Drug Take-Back Day events.

  https://www.deadiversion.usdoj.gov/drug_disposal/takeback/

  DEA-registered collector for prescription drugs and dietary supplements.

  https://apps2.deadiversion.usdoj.gov/pubdispsearch/spring/main?execution=e1s1

  A community prescription drug or dietary supplement collector.

  https://www.deadiversion.usdoj.gov/drug_disposal/index.html

REFERENCES

Akoglu, B., Schrott, M., Bolouri, H., Jaffari, A., Kutschera, E., Caspary, W.F., & Faust, D. (2008). The folic acid metabolite L-5-methyltetrahydrofolate effectively reduced total serum homocysteine level in orthotopic liver transplant recipients: a double-blind placebo-controlled study. *European Journal of Clinical Nutrition, 62*, 796–801. PMID: 17522618.

Asher, G.N., Corbett, A.H., & Hawke, R.L. (2017). Common herbal dietary supplement-drug interactions. *American Family Physician, 96*(2), 101–107. https://www.ncbi.nlm.nih.gov/pubmed/28762712. PMID: 28762712.

Boden, W.E., Bhatt, D.L, Toth, P.P., et al. (2020). Profound reductions in first and total cardiovascular events with icosapent ethyl in the REDUCE-IT trial: Why these results usher in a new era in dyslipidaemia therapeutics. *European Heart Journal, 41*(24), 2304–12.

Brotanek, J.M., Gosz, J., Weitzman, M., & Flores, G. (2007). Iron deficiency in early childhood in the United States: Risk factors and racial/ethnic disparities. *Pediatrics, 120*, 568–75. PMID: 17766530.

Cooperman, T. (2020, April 25). *Multivitamin and multimineral supplements review.* ConsumerLab. https://www.consumerlab.com/reviews/multivitamin_review_comparisons/multivitamins/

Del Gobbo, L.C., Imamura, F., Aslibekyan, S., Marklund, M., Virtanen, J.K., Wennberg, M., et al. (2016). Omega-3 polyunsaturated fatty acid biomarkers and coronary heart disease: pooling project of 19 cohort studies. *JAMA Internal Medicine, 176*, 1155–66.

Flock, M.R., Skulas-Ray, A.C., Harris, W.S, Etherton, T.D, Fleming, J.A., & Kris-Etherton, P.M. (2013). Determinants of erythrocyte omega-3 fatty acid content in response to fish oil supplementation: a dose-response randomized controlled trial. *Journal of the American Heart Association, 2*(6), e000513. PMID: 24252845.

Food and Drug Administration. (2017, November 28). *The FDA warns that biotin may interfere with lab tests: FDA safety communication.* Department of Health and Human Services, Food and Drug Administration.

Food and Drug Administration. (2019, June 19). *FDA announces new qualified health claims for EPA and DHA omega-3 consumption and the risk of hypertension and coronary heart disease.* Department of Health and Human Services, Food and Drug Administration.

Gardiner, P., Phillips, R., & Shaughnessy, A.F. (2008). Herbal and dietary supplement-drug interactions in patients with chronic illnesses. *American Family Physician, 77*(1), 73–78. PMID: 18236826.

Geller, A.I., Shehab, N., Weidle, N.J., Lovegrove, M.C., Wolpert, B.J., Timbo, B.B., Mozersky, R.P., & Budnitz, D.S. (2015). Emergency department visits for adverse events related to dietary supplements. *The New England Journal of Medicine, 373*(16), 1531–40. PMID: 26465986.

Holick, M.F., Binkley, N.C., Bischoff-Ferrari, H.A., Gordon, C.M., Hanley, D.A., Heaney, R.P., Murad, M.H., Weaver, C.M., Endocrine Society. (2011). Evaluation, treatment and prevention of vitamin D deficiency: an Endocrine Society clinical practice guideline. *Journal of Clinical Endocrinology and Metabolism, 96*(7), 1911–30. PMID: 21646368.

Hu, Y., Hu, F.B., & Manson, J.E. (2019). Marine omega-3 supplementation and cardiovascular disease: An updated meta-analysis of 13 randomized controlled trials involving 127 477 participants. *Journal of the American Heart Association, 8,* e013543

Institute of Medicine, Food and Nutrition Board. (2010). *Dietary Reference Intakes for Calcium and Vitamin D.* National Academy Press.

Institute of Medicine, Food and Nutrition Board. (2001) *Dietary Reference Intakes for Vitamin A, Vitamin K, Arsenic, Boron, Chromium, Copper, Iodine, Iron, Manganese, Molybdenum, Nickel, Silicon, Vanadium, and Zinc.* National Academy Press.

Manson, J.E., Cook, N.R.. Lee, I., Christen, W., Bassuk, S.S., Mora, S., Gibson, H., Gordon, D., Copeland, T., D'Agostino, D., Friedenberg,

G., Ridge, C., Bubes, V., Giovannucci, E.L., Willett, W.C., & Buring, J.E. (VITAL Research Group). (2019). Vitamin D supplements and prevention of cancer and cardiovascular disease. *New England Journal of Medicine, 380*(1), 33–44. PMID: 30415629.

Mayo Foundation for Medical Education and Research. (2018a). *Vitamin deficiency anemia.* Mayo Clinic. https://www.mayoclinic.org /diseases-conditions/vitamin-deficiency-anemia/diagnosis-treatment /drc-20355031

———. (2018b). *Warfarin side effects: Watch for interactions.* Mayo Clinic. https://www.mayoclinic.org/diseases-conditions/deep-vein -thrombosis/in-depth/warfarin-side-effects/art-20047592

Mazereeuw, G., Lanctot, K.L., Chau, S.A., Swardfager, W., & Herrmann, N. (2012). Effects of omega-3 fatty acids on cognitive performance: A meta-analysis. *Neurobiology of Aging, 33*(7), 1482 e17–29. PMID: 22305186.

Mei, Z., Cogswell, M.E., Looker, A.C., Pfeiffer, C.M., Cusick, S.E., Lacher, D.A., et al. (2011). Assessment of iron status in US pregnant women from the National Health and Nutrition Examination Survey (NHANES), 1999–2006. *American Journal of Clinical Nutrition, 93*, 1312–20. PMID: 21430118.

National Institutes of Health. (2018). *Iron.* U.S. Department of Health and Human Services, National Institutes of Health. https:// ods.od.nih.gov/factsheets/Iron-HealthProfessional/

National Institutes of Health, Office of Dietary Supplements (2020). *Vitamin D-Fact Sheet for Consumers.* https://ods.od.nih.gov /factsheets/VitaminD-health%20Professional/#en12

National Institute of Health. Office of Dietary Supplements Dietary Supplements Fact Sheets. Accessed February 2021. https:// ods.od.nih.gov/factsheets/list-all/

National Research Council (US) Committee on Diet and Health. (1989). Trace elements. In *Diet and Health: Implications for Reducing Chronic Disease Risk.* (pp. 367–412). National Academies Press (US).

Rocha, T., Amaral, J., & Oliveira, M. (2015). Adulteration of dietary supplements by the illegal addition of synthetic drugs: A review. *Comprehensive Reviews in Food Science and Food Safety, 15*(1), 43–62. https://onlinelibrary.wiley.com/doi/abs/10.1111/1541-4337.12173

Rosenbloom, M. (2020, June 1). *Vitamin toxicity.* Medscape. https://emedicine.medscape.com/article/819426-overview#a4

Troen, A.M., Mitchell, B., Sorensen, B., et al. (2006). Unmetabolized folic acid in plasma is associated with reduced natural killer cell cytotoxicity among postmenopausal women. *Journal of Nutrition, 136,* 189–94. PMID: 16365081.

United States Preventive Services Task Force. (2021, April 13). *Final recommendation statement: Vitamin D deficiency in Adults: Screening.* United States Preventive Services Task Force. https://www.uspreventiveservicestaskforce.org/uspstf/recommendation/vitamin-d-deficiency-screening

https://www.uspreventiveservicestaskforce.org/uspstf/recommendation/vitamin-d-deficiency-screening

United States Preventive Services Task Force (2018). Vitamin D, Calcium, or combined supplementation for the primary prevention of fractures in community-dwelling adults: US Preventive Services Task Force Recommendation Statement. *JAMA,* 319(15), 1592–1599. PMID: 29677309.

Zeratsky, K. (2020, April 17). *What is vitamin D toxicity?* Mayo Clinic Healthy Lifestyle: Nutrition and Healthy Eating. https://www.mayoclinic.org/healthy-lifestyle/nutrition-and-healthy-eating/expert-answers/vitamin-d-toxicity/faq-20058108

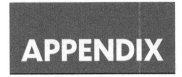

DIETARY SUPPLEMENTS AND COVID-19

Since the beginning of the COVID-19 pandemic, I have received a deluge of questions from people who would like to know which dietary supplements they should take to prevent being infected by the coronavirus. People have asked me how much zinc, elderberry, or vitamin C they should take to boost their immune system. Some friends have even asked me if taking high doses of vitamin C would make them so immune to infection that they would not need to wear a mask. The majority of these questions start with a simple statement like "I read on the internet (blogs, social media, etc.) that taking elderberry would boost my immune system or it would kill the virus." One person asked me if she should take colloidal silver at a much higher dose than she usually takes. I told her absolutely not, then proceeded to share all of the side effects of a colloidal silver overdose, or any dose. While an uptick in dietary supplement usage or dosage may not seem significant, the lack of knowledge and misinformation around the pandemic are a significant cause for concern. In recent months, the sales of dietary supplements have surged nationwide (and worldwide) as scared consumers view what they see on TV commercials, blogs, and social media posts as scientific evidence in support of using dietary supplements. However, when it comes to the underlying science about this novel coronavirus, much still needs to be learned.

For those who might be too busy or do not want to read this section in detail, below is the abridged version of my response to these questions:

There is insufficient evidence supporting a therapeutic role for any dietary supplements to prevent or treat COVID-19, and using dietary supplements in high doses can be harmful. If you have low levels of vitamin D, I recommend that you take a vitamin D supplement, get safe sun exposure, and eat foods rich in vitamin D. For now, to boost your immune system, I recommend that you eat a nutritious diet rich in fresh (or frozen) fruits and vegetables, get at least seven to eight hours of sleep per night, exercise, and manage your stress.

For those who are interested in learning more about the efficacy and safety of dietary supplements in the context of COVID-19, this section highlights some immune-related compounds that many have been asking about. While not exhaustive, this section seeks to give you a better understanding of the current science about using dietary supplements to prevent COVID-19.

Since the onset of the COVID-19 pandemic, sales of dietary supplements have skyrocketed worldwide, especially the ones with claims to boost the immune system. Sales of supplements such as elderberry, zinc, vitamin C, and echinacea increased by 415%, 255%, 146%, and 122% respectively in the week ending March 8, 2020 (Information Resources Inc., 2021). While these drastic increases might seem like typographical errors, market research suggests that this was simply the start of an upward trend, as people around the world have sought ways to combat the spread of the virus (Information Resources Inc., 2021). The nutritional supplement industry in the United States saw a net gain of $345 million in 2019. During the first six weeks of the coronavirus pandemic (until April 5, 2020), sales of nutritional supplements experienced a net gain of $435 million, and in the following six weeks (until May 17, 2020), sales of these supplements gained another $151 million. In recent months, these sales rates have begun leveling off, but when compared to previous years, the net gains are still significantly higher. For instance, sale of vitamins appears to be higher by 16% in 2020, when compared to 2019. The rate of increase is more than three times what it was in 2019, when sales surpassed those of 2018 by only 5% (Information Resources Inc., 2021; SPINS, 2021).

There is no doubt that we are all panicked, and we tend to buy dietary supplements based on emotional decisions and not logical ones. There are several reasons for this increase in sales, but the driving force appears to be unproven claims by medical entertainment personalities and dietary supplement manufacturers on television programs and social media platforms. They promote the use of dietary supplements such as vitamin C, elderberry, zinc, and vitamin D to either prevent or cure COVID-19. And with limited scientific evidence available on COVID-19, as research is ongoing, misinformation has been able to spread across the worldwide web, creating what the World Health Organization refers to as an "infodemic" (World Health Organization, 2020). Analyses of Google trends have revealed that searches for dietary supplements, herbs, and other bioactive compounds experienced a sharp uptick at the height of the pandemic, when global quarantine efforts were well underway (Hamulka et al., 2021). However, interest in particular compounds have waxed and waned, as trends have brought each into focus for their general immune-boosting or antiviral properties (Hamulka et al., 2021).

Let's talk about a few commonly used dietary supplements that have been heavily marketed for the management of COVID-19. In some of the marketing campaign of these supplements, we see phrases such as "proven scientifically" or "been shown scientifically to kill the novel coronavirus that causes COVID-19." To better understand the underlying science, and the gap that is not often addressed in this language, please review chapter 4 (The Science of Dietary Supplements) in this book. While these phrases make it sound like sufficient evidence exists, the results of an experiment in a petri dish that discovered that elderberry exhibited antiviral activity against human coronavirus cannot be extrapolated to COVID-19. And anecdotal reports from a few people who took elderberry and did not get COVID-19 do not constitute scientific evidence either.

Science takes vast amounts of time and resources to come to reliable and reproducible results. During a rapidly-changing public health crisis like the COVID-19 pandemic, the time required to come to scientific conclusions can seem extraordinary. But this allows scientists, healthcare professionals, and the general public to make informed decisions. So, as always, before you start taking any dietary supplements, talk to your physician or healthcare provider to make sure that you are taking the correct dose and that they are not interacting with other drugs that you may be taking. Although we are still learning every day about diseases like COVID-19, we already have some basic knowledge about how some dietary supplements such as vitamins work. Let's take a look at some of the most widely discussed supplements over the course of the pandemic.

VITAMIN D

The scientific studies that evaluated the efficacy of vitamin D for COVID-19 point in a common direction: Vitamin D deficiency may make people more prone to become infected and develop COVID-19 (Adams et al., 2020). Some reports suggested that administration of vitamin D to patients with COVID-19 who are hospitalized can shorten the length of hospital stay, but as of now, randomized trials have not proven that these reports are accurate (Hernández et al., 2020; Ohaegbulam et al., 2020). My recommendation is that you check your 25-hydroxyvitamin D levels. If they are less than 25 nmol/L, then you need to take vitamin D supplements. Consumption of high doses of vitamin D (often in excess of 4000 IU per day) can result in adverse effects including high levels of calcium, so it's important to monitor your intake.

VITAMIN C

Clinical trials on the use of vitamin C in common cold collectively suggest that regular use of vitamin C can shorten the duration of the common cold by 8% (Hemilä & Chalker, 2013). However, we cannot extrapolate the results of these studies to COVID-19 because

COVID-19 is caused by a novel coronavirus that is genetically different from the coronavirus that causes the common cold (Wang et al., 2020). There are a number of claims on the effectiveness of high-dose vitamin C, both orally and intravenously, but at the time of this writing there is no scientific evidence to prove that vitamin C can be taken to prevent or treat COVID-19. In a randomized clinical trial that tested the effectiveness of a daily intake of high-dose zinc (50 mg), vitamin C (8000 mg), both agents, or standard of care for ten days in ambulatory patients with COVID-19, it was reported that neither zinc, vitamin C, nor their combination significantly decreased the duration of the symptoms associated with COVID-19 (Thomas et al., 2021). I recommend that you consume vitamin C–rich fruits and vegetables to have adequate intake of vitamin C. High doses of vitamin C may result in gastrointestinal side effects such as nausea, vomiting, heartburn, and diarrhea and can also cause the formation of kidney stones.

ZINC

Zinc has been promoted to treat and prevent the common cold, although the results of studies (most of them with low-quality methodologies) that evaluated the impact of zinc on the common cold are conflicting. One of the most comprehensive systemic reviews of clinical studies on zinc concluded that zinc supplementation may reduce the duration of the common cold by 1.65 days (Science et al., 2012). However, when it comes to COVID-19, a recent retrospective analysis showed that there was no association between supplementation with zinc and survival in hospitalized patients with COVID-19 (Yao et al., 2020). This study was retrospective and the zinc levels were not measured, and some critics indicated that measuring the zinc levels of the patients who received zinc supplementation would have resulted in a different conclusion (Khurana et al., 2021). Although zinc at oral doses below 40 mg/day is considered safe, higher doses can result in gastrointestinal adverse events and loss of taste. Zinc should never be used nasally because it may result in permanent loss of taste (Jafek et al., 2004).

ELDERBERRY

Elderberry is reported to have antiviral properties due to its ability to modulate inflammation (Thomas et al., 2020). However, the results of clinical studies on the efficacy of elderberry to prevent or treat the common cold are conflicting (Mahboubi, 2020). This is mostly due to the low quality of such studies, which include small sample sizes and lack of sound statistical analyses, and the fact that most of these studies were funded by the companies that sell elderberry products (Hint: Conflict of interest!). Although elderberry is derived from a naturally-occurring plant (*Sambucus nigra*), and the general public believes that plant-based products are largely safe, science suggests otherwise. Patients with diabetes should refrain from taking elderberry because it can interfere with insulin secretion and glucose metabolism. It has also been reported that elderberry can result in a number of cardiovascular side effects, such as low blood pressure and tachycardia (an increase in heart rate) (Ulbricht et al., 2014). Elderberry can also cause dehydration and low levels of potassium due to diuresis and can interfere with prescription drugs such as immunosuppressants (Ulbricht et al., 2014).

SILVER

In 1999, the FDA issued warnings that over-the-counter products that contain silver and colloidal silver were unsafe and misbranded (FDA, 1999). Despite these warnings, colloidal silver is still widely available and is now heavily marketed as a potential preventive therapy and cure for COVID-19. The most common side effect of silver is argyria, a grayish skin discoloration that is permanent (Chung et al., 2010). Silver can also cause other serious side effects such as neurotoxicity, blood cancer, and liver and kidney disease (Keung et al., 2020).

Given the significant prevalence of side effects and the guidance of the FDA, please DO NOT TAKE any dietary supplements that contain silver or colloidal silver.

CONCLUSION

While marketing campaigns and misinformation prevalent on social media platforms would suggest otherwise, the best method for prevention of COVID-19 (as with most infectious diseases) is to avoid being exposed to the virus that causes the disease. Rather than taking nutritional supplements, herbal remedies, or treatments, follow the Centers for Disease Control and Prevention (CDC) recommendations to wear a mask over the nose and mouth in public, and to avoid touching the face with unwashed hands. The CDC also recommends avoiding contact with people who have COVID-19 and to practice social distancing.

The only scientifically proven interventions to boost the immune system are to eat a nutritious diet rich in fruits and vegetables, get adequate sleep, exercise regularly, and manage your stress. A number of companies, wellness enthusiasts, celebrities, TV personalities, and social media influencers have preyed on public anxiety and fears during the COVID-19 pandemic. The FDA and Federal Trade Commission have sent letters to many companies warning them to stop advertising fraudulent therapies to prevent or treat COVID-19 (FDA Office of Regulatory Affairs, 2021). Although these federal agencies make their best efforts to monitor websites and social media platforms to identify fraudulent claims, at the end of the day it is our responsibility as consumers to make informed decisions. This means relying on high-quality scientific evidence. It is important to critically examine, investigate, and research claims before taking nutritional supplements or sharing these suggestions with others.

ADDITIONAL RESOURCES

- Fraudulent coronavirus disease 2019 (COVID-19) products/ List of companies with fraudulent claims.

  https://www.fda.gov/consumers/health-fraud-scams /fraudulent-coronavirus-disease-2019-covid-19-products

- Centers for Disease Control and Prevention, Coronavirus (COVID-19)

  https://www.cdc.gov/coronavirus/2019-ncov/index.html

- ClinicalTrials.gov, Clinical studies related to COVID-19

  https://clinicaltrials.gov/ct2/results?cond=COVID-19

- Infectious Diseases Society of America, COVID-19 Resource Center

  https://www.idsociety.org/public-health/COVID-19

- National Institutes of Health, Coronavirus (COVID-19)

  https://www.nih.gov/health-information/coronavirus

- National Institutes of Health, Office of Dietary Supplements

  https://ods.od.nih.gov

REFERENCES

Adams, K. K., Baker, W. L., & Sobieraj, D. M. (2020). Myth busters: Dietary supplements and COVID-19. *The Annals of Pharmacotherapy*, *54*(8), 820–826.

Chung, I.-S., Lee, M.-Y., Shin, D.-H., & Jung, H.-R. (2010). Three systemic argyria cases after ingestion of colloidal silver solution. *International Journal of Dermatology*, *49*(10), 1175–1177.

FDA Office of Regulatory Affairs. (2021). *Fraudulent coronavirus disease 2019 (COVID-19) products*. FDA. https://www.fda.gov/consumers/health-fraud-scams/fraudulent-coronavirus-disease-2019-covid-19-products

Food & Drug Administration. (1999). Over-the-counter drug products containing colloidal silver ingredients or silver salts. *Public Health Service (PHS), Food and Drug Administration (FDA): Final Rule*. Fed Regist, 64, 44653–44658.

Hamulka, J., Jeruszka-Bielak, M., Górnicka, M., Drywień, M. E., & Zielinska-Pukos, M. A. (2021). Dietary supplements during COVID-19 outbreak. Results of Google trends analysis supported by PLifeCOVID-19 online studies. *Nutrients*, *13*(1), 54.

Hemilä, H., & Chalker, E. (2013). Vitamin C for preventing and treating the common cold. *Cochrane Database of Systematic Reviews, 1*.

Hernández, J. L., Nan, D., Fernandez-Ayala, M., García-Unzueta, M., Hernández-Hernández, M. A., López-Hoyos, M., Muñoz-Cacho, P., Olmos, J. M., Gutiérrez-Cuadra, M., & Ruiz-Cubillán, J. J. (2020). Vitamin D status in hospitalized patients with SARS-CoV-2 infection. *The Journal of Clinical Endocrinology and Metabolism*, 106(3), e1343-e1353.

Information Resources Inc. (2021). *IRI | Delivering Growth for CPG, Retail, and Healthcare*. https://www.iriworldwide.com/en-us

Jafek, B. W., Linschoten, M. R., & Murrow, B. W. (2004). Anosmia after intranasal zinc gluconate use. *American Journal of Rhinology*, *18*(3), 137–141.

Johnstone, J., Roth, D. E., Gordon Guyatt, M. D., & Mark Loeb, M. D. (2012). Zinc for the treatment of the common cold: A systematic review and meta-analysis of randomized controlled trials. *Canadian Medical Association Journal, 184*(10), E551.

Keung, Y.-K., Wang, T., & Hong-Lung Hu, E. (2020). Acute myeloid leukemia with complex cytogenetic abnormalities associated with long-term use of oral colloidal silver as nutritional supplement–Case report and review of literature. *Journal of Oncology Pharmacy Practice, 26*(1), 212–215.

Khurana, A. K., Karna, S. T., & Hussain, A. (2021). Zinc and coronavirus disease 2019: Causal or casual association? *Chest, 159*(1), 449–450.

Mahboubi, M. (2020, July 10). *Sambucus nigra* (black elder) as alternative treatment for cold and flu. *Advances in Traditional Medicine, 1*–10.

Ohaegbulam, K. C., Swalih, M., Patel, P., Smith, M. A., & Perrin, R. (2020). Vitamin D supplementation in COVID-19 patients: A clinical case series. *American Journal of Therapeutics*, e485.

Science, M., Johnstone, J., Roth, D. E., Guyatt, G., & Loeb, M. (2012). Zinc for the treatment of the common cold: A systematic review and meta-analysis of randomized controlled trials. *Canadian Medical Association Journal, 184*(10), E551–E561.

SPINS. (2021). *SPINS: A wellness-focused data technology company.* SPINS. https://www.spins.com/

Thomas, A. L., Byers, P. L., Vincent, P. L., & Applequist, W. L. (2020). Medicinal attributes of American elderberry. In *Medicinal and Aromatic Plants of North America* (pp. 119–139). Springer.

Thomas, S., Patel, D., Bittel, B., Wolski, K., Wang, Q., Kumar, A., Il'Giovine, Z.J., Mehra, R., McWilliams, C., Nissen, S.E., & Desai, M.Y. Effect of high-dose zinc and ascorbic acid supplementation vs usual care on symptom length and reduction among ambulatory patients with SARS-CoV-2 infection: The COVID A to Z randomized clinical trial. *JAMA Netw Open*, 2021 Feb 1;4(2): e210369. doj:10.1001/jamanetworkopen.2021.0369.PMID:33576820.

Ulbricht, C., Basch, E., Cheung, L., Goldberg, H., Hammerness, P., Isaac, R., Khalsa, K. P. S., Romm, A., Rychlik, I., & Varghese, M. (2014). An evidence-based systematic review of elderberry and elderflower (*Sambucus nigra*) by the Natural Standard Research Collaboration. *Journal of Dietary Supplements, 11*(1), 80–120.

Wang, L., Wang, Y., Ye, D., & Liu, Q. (2020). Review of the 2019 novel coronavirus (SARS-CoV-2) based on current evidence. *International Journal of Antimicrobial Agents, 55*(6), 105948. https://doi.org/10.1016/j.ijantimicag.2020.105948

World Health Organization. (2020). *Managing the COVID-19 infodemic: Promoting healthy behaviours and mitigating the harm from misinformation and disinformation.* World Health Organization. https://www.who.int/news/item/23-09-2020-managing-the-covid-19-infodemic-promoting-healthy-behaviours-and-mitigating-the-harm-from-misinformation-and-disinformation

Yao, J. S., Paguio, J. A., Dee, E. C., Tan, H. C., Moulick, A., Milazzo, C., Jurado, J., Della Penna, N., & Celi, L. A. (2020). The minimal effect of zinc on the survival of hospitalized patients with Covid-19: An observational study. *Chest, 159*(1), 108–111.

THANK YOU

Thank you so much for investing your time reading through my book. I hope it has inspired you to make informed decisions when it comes to choosing the dietary supplements needed to enhance your health. Please take just a moment to share your thoughts in a review wherever you purchased this book. Readers rely on honest, thoughtful feedback from the wider community to help them make more informed decisions. It also helps me as an author refine my message and deliver relevant information and content my readers need. I read each review personally and appreciate your honest feedback.

Don't forget to sign up for my blog on www.mahtabjafari.com

Sincerely,

Mahtab Jafari

ABOUT THE AUTHOR

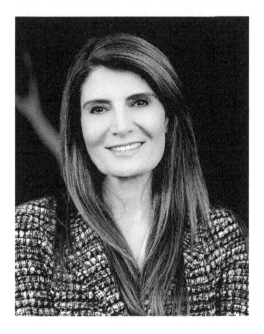

Mahtab Jafari is a Professor of Pharmaceutical Sciences and the director of the UCI Center for Healthspan Sciences at the University of California, Irvine. Her research focuses on slowing the aging process and adding healthy years to human life through a science that she introduced—Healthspan Pharmacology. Dr. Jafari is passionate about educating and inspiring her students and the community to adopt a healthy lifestyle. Her popular course, *Life101: Mental and Physical Self-Care*, is offered on www.coursera.org.

Made in the USA
Coppell, TX
07 September 2021

61984136R00108